Vita-Guard Keto For Everyone Revised

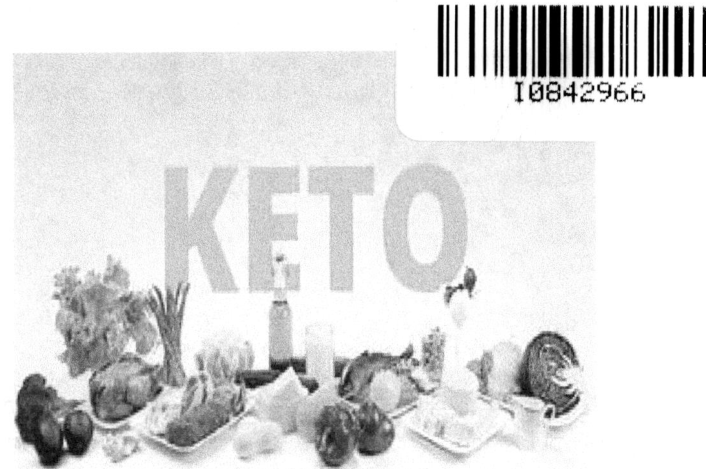

Published by

Vita-Guard

Email: vitaguardKeto1912@gmail.com

Foreword

Who Needs Keto Diet?

In short, everyone needs to be on the Keto diet. The Keto diet is not just for weight loss. It will help you to convert to a healthy body and avoid many diseases.

Benefits of a Ketogenic Diet

There are numerous benefits that come with being on keto: from weight loss and increased energy levels to therapeutic medical applications. Most anyone can safely benefit from eating a low-carb, high-fat diet. Below, you'll find a short list of the benefits you can receive from a ketogenic diet.

Below are some of the reasons everyone needs the keto diet:

Weight Loss

The ketogenic diet essentially uses your body fat as an energy source – so there are obvious weight loss benefits. On keto, your insulin (the fat storing hormone) levels drop greatly which turns your body into a fat burning machine.

Scientifically, the ketogenic diet has **shown better results** compared to low-fat and high-carb diets; even in the long term.

Many people incorporate MCT Oil into their diet (it increases ketone production and fat loss) by drinking **keto proof coffee** in the morning

Control Blood Sugar

Keto naturally lowers blood sugar levels due to the type of foods you eat. Studies even show that the ketogenic diet is a **more effective** way to manage and prevent diabetes compared to low-calorie diets.

If you're pre-diabetic or have Type II diabetes, you should seriously consider a ketogenic diet. We have many readers that have had success with their blood sugar control on keto.

Mental Focus

Many people use the ketogenic diet *specifically* for the increased mental performance.

Ketones are a great source of fuel for the brain. When you lower carb intake, you avoid big spikes in blood sugar. Together, this can result in improved focus and concentration .

Studies show that an increased intake of fatty acids can have impacting benefits to our brain's function.

Increased Energy & Normalized Hunger

By giving your body a better and more reliable energy source, you will feel more energized during the day. Fats are shown to be the most effective molecule to burn as fuel.

On top of that, fat is naturally more satisfying and ends up leaving us in a satiated ("full") state for longer.

Epilepsy

The ketogenic diet has been used since the early 1900's to treat epilepsy successfully. It is still one of the most widely used therapies for children who have uncontrolled epilepsy today.

One of the main benefits of the ketogenic diet and epilepsy

is that it allows fewer medications to be used while still offering excellent control.

In the last few years, studies have also shown significant results in adults treated with keto as well.

Cholesterol & Blood Pressure

A keto diet has shown to improve triglyceride levels and cholesterol levels most associated with arterial buildup. More specifically low-carb, high-fat diets show a dramatic increase in HDL and decrease in LDL particle concentration compared to low-fat diets.

Many studies on low-carb diets also show better improvement in blood pressure over other diets.

Some blood pressure issues are associated with excess weight, which is a bonus since keto tends to lead to weight loss. If you have high blood pressure or other blood pressure issues.

Insulin Resistance

Insulin resistance can lead to type II diabetes if left unmanaged. An abundant amount of research shows that a low carb, ketogenic diet can help people lower their insulin levels to healthy ranges.

Even if you're athletic, you can benefit from insulin optimization on keto through eating foods high in omega-3 fatty acids,

Acne

It's common to experience improvements in your skin when you switch to a ketogenic diet.

A study that shows drops in lesions and skin inflammation when switching to a low-carb diet. Another study that shows a probable connection between high-carb eating and increased acne, so it's likely that keto can help.

For acne, it may be beneficial to reduce dairy intake and

follow a strict skin cleaning regimen.

Before and After Pictures of People who lost Weight on the Keto Diet

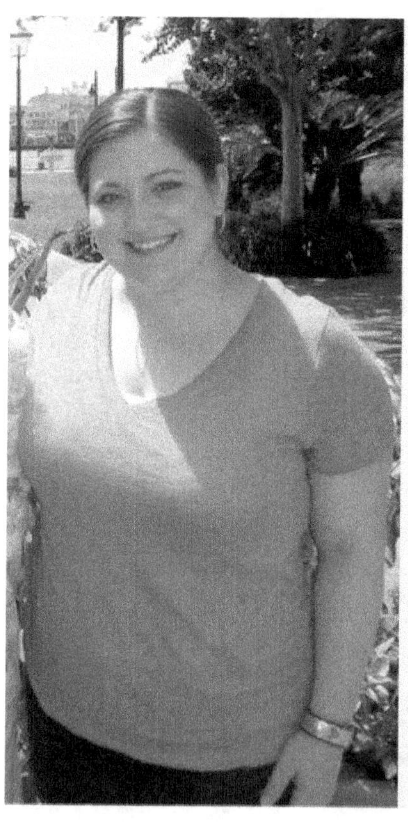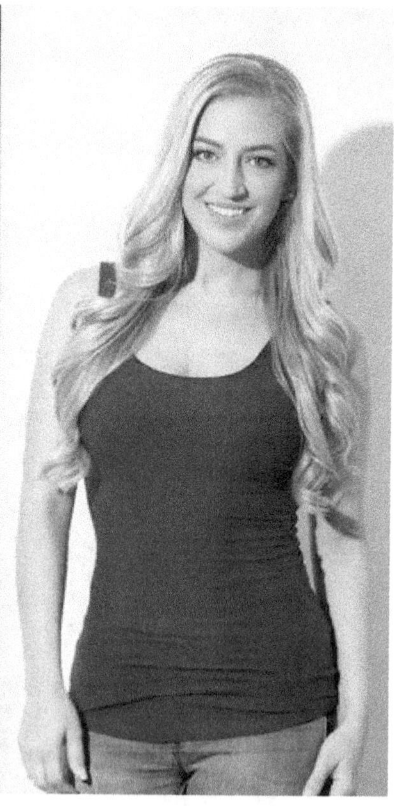

Chapter One

About Ketosis

Shopping for Keto foods can be very frustrating for some people. When you read articles on Google about Keto foods, many of the foods listed are seldom known by most shoppers.

This book was written for the purpose of simplifying shopping for the right and better know Keto foods. Avoid going out and loading your pantry with all the foods listed in the book. Make a slow change-over. Should there be foods that you are not accustom to eating, buy a small amount and train yourself to acquire the taste.

What is ketosis?

Ketosis is a metabolic state in which some of the body's energy supply comes from ketone bodies in the blood, in contrast to a state of glycolysis in which blood glucose provides energy. Generally, ketosis occurs when the body is metabolizing fat at a high rate and converting fatty acids into ketones.

WHAT ARE THE BENEFITS OF THE KETO DIET?

- Aids In Weight Loss

- Slow Down The Aging Process

- Improve GI Performance and Digestion

- Increase Daily Energy

- Decreases Inflammation Which Improves Acne, Arthri-

  tis, IBS and more)

- Improve Cognitive Function

- Improves Sleep

- Increase Mental Clarity (increases memory, cognition

  and clarity)

- Improve Daily Performance

- Fights Cancer

- Prevents Heart Disease

- And Much More!

So, we should conclude that the Keto diet is for everyone who wants a healthy body.

Before and After Pictures of People who lost Weight on the Keto Diet

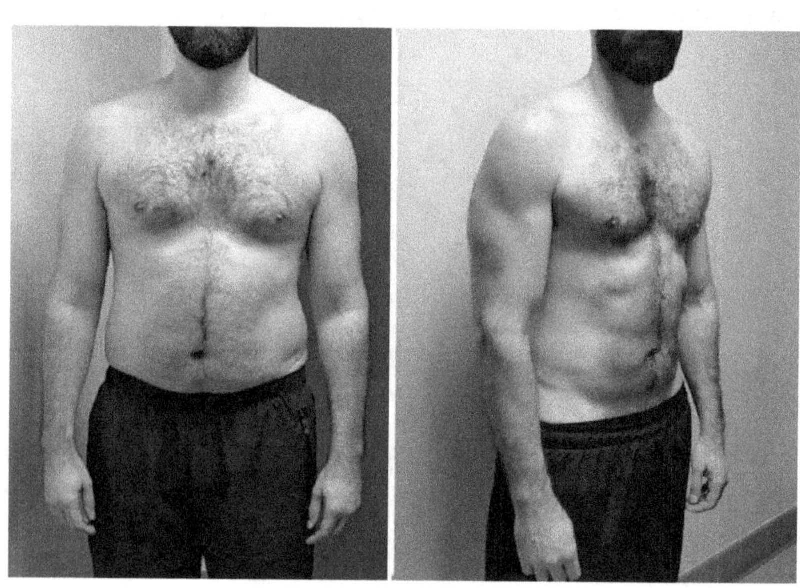

Chapter Two

How To Almost Instantly Get Into Ketosis With The Help Of A Few Tricks

Nowadays, there are tons of diets that seem promising when it comes to shredding fat. However, only a small number of them actually live up to our expectations and get us the results we want after the first week or two. This is the same reason why many people have second thoughts about diets and cannot crack the code behind the perfect weight loss program.

However, if there is a single diet that has shown massive results to many people across the globe, it has to be the ketogenic diet. In case you have never heard about it... The Ketogenic Diet is basically a way of making your body function on a very low-carb eating regimen that shares many similarities with the famous Atkins and other low-carb diets.

Basically, the diet forces the body to enter a state known as 'ketosis' which actually means that it is using fat as its main fuel instead of the carbohydrate intake. The Ketogenic Diet Benefits of The Keto Diet The benefits of the Keto Diet are endless. According to a lot of studies and reviews, the diet is proven to:

- Kill your appetite - The automatic reduction in appetite lets you eat more protein and carbs and therefore consume much fewer calories

- Boost your weight loss - Studies have shown that people on low-carb diets lose more weight faster than ones doing the low-fat diets

- Shred the abdominal area - Knowing that not all fat body is the same, the keto diet is based on shredding the abdominal area and the subcutaneous fat (located under the skin) and then the visceral fat (in the abdominal cavity), reducing all the harmful abdominal fat

- Lower the triglyceride levels (prevents heart disease) - Also known as fat molecules, the triglycerides are naturally occurring in our body - but can be significantly lowered with the keto diet and with that lower the risk of heart disease.

- Increase levels of HDL levels (the 'good' cholesterol) - The High Density Lipoprotein (HDL) commonly known as the 'good cholesterol' is drastically increased in the blood, helping the body reuse or excrete them if needed and with that again lowering the risk of heart disease.

- Reduce the blood sugar and insulin levels - Carbs are broken down into simple sugars when digested. With a low-carb diet, this process is put to an end and the bloodstream is not full of blood sugar.

- Lower the blood pressure - Reducing carbs leads to a significant reduction in blood pressure which also links to a reduced risk of many common diseases

- Treat the metabolic syndrome - People with abdominal obesity, elevated blood pressure, high triglycerides and low HDL levels can all benefit from the Keto Diet which boosts their metabolism and prevents a lot of diseases.

- Help with brain disorders - Glucose is known as necessary for the brain, which is certainly true. However, a large part of our brain can also burn ketones, which are formed during starvation or when the intake of carbs is low.

- Lower the blood pressure - Reducing carbs leads to a significant reduction in blood pressure which also links to a reduced risk of many common diseases

- Treat the metabolic syndrome - People with abdominal obesity, elevated blood pressure, high triglycerides and low HDL levels can all benefit from the Keto Diet which boosts their metabolism and prevents a lot of diseases.

- Help with brain disorders - Glucose is known as necessary for the brain, which is certainly true. However, a large part of our brain can also burn ketones, which are formed during starvation or when the intake of carbs is low.

Why Entering The State of Ketosis Is Important Going into the state of ketosis means shifting from a carbohydrate to a fat intake, making your body burn fat instead of carbohydrates.

Wondering why? Well, when we eat carbs, our body uses (most of) them to burn energy. However, the residue of carbs is stored and glucose and usually converted to fat. This is why most people cannot lose weight even though they exercise on a regular basis. Scientifically, the Keto Diet is proven to work and has shown great results for many people over the years. However, getting used to it is often the big problem that people are facing from the very start. From nausea to anxiousness and sometimes loss of energy, the 'keto flu' is a part of the beginning phases of ketosis.

Fat Fasting The Main Focus of The Keto Diet Fat fasting is what makes the keto diet work. In a nutshell, it is directly linked with entering the state of ketosis quickly. What it bases on is eating as much fat as you can so that your body adapts to your fat intake rather than the carb intake. Even though the name may not sound right to you (considering the fact that it means eating a lot of fats), it is a proven natural way to get into ketosis fast.

Before and After Pictures of People who lost Weight on the Keto Diet

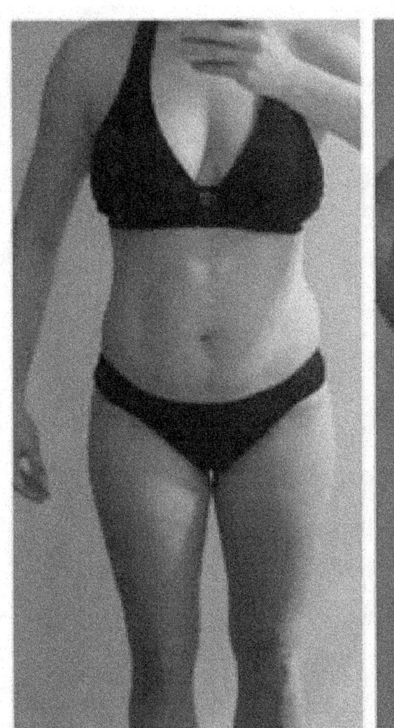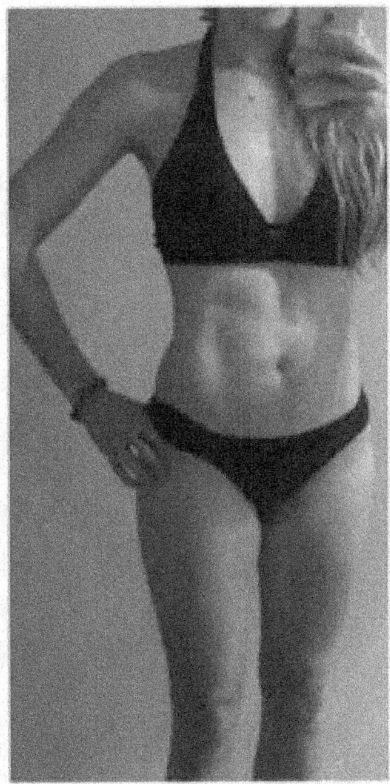

Chapter Three

Vita-Guard Keto Tricks to Enter

a State of Ketosis

Vita-Guard Keto Trick #1 - The first way to hack the Keto-genic diet and enter the state of ketosis earlier than expected is to take Vita-Guard Keto. This product is from Vita-Guard Keto, 91 E. Main Street, Inman, SC 29349. The cost is $39.95 for a 30 day supply. The shipping is free.

See website for special savings on shipping.

You earn cash back which will provide you with extra income.

Vita-Guard Keto Trick # 2 - Limit your intake of carbohydrates to 35—50 grams per day. Remember the key to the Keto diet is Low carbs, limited proteins and high in fats. On the surface this contradicts what we have been taught.

Vita-Guard Keto Trick # 3 - You can eat an unlimited amount of cheese, provided you choose the right cheese. Avoid creamy cheese in a tube. Choose a cheese with zero carbohydrates. There are many ways you can eat cheese. Put grated cheese on scrambled eggs. Avoid the shredded cheese bought in the market. It has been coated with substance to keep it fresh that is taboo on a Keto diet. Buy the block cheese and grate it yourself.

A great snack when you get hungry is to eat a piece of brie cheese or Babybel cheeses. Babybel cheese is good to have around when you are away from home as they last long outside the fridge and is good packed and can easily be included in the bag. Always select cheeses with as high-fat as possible.

There are those who limit their intake of dairy

products including cheese and then they see that it inhibits weight loss. Others have no problems at all with eating cheese – it varies and you have yourself come up with what is an appropriate level. It is not the carbohydrates in the cheese that inhibit weight loss since there is often not a high amount of carbohydrates in cheese. Usually instead it is the milk protein in cheese that is the culprit.

Vita-Guard Keto Trick # 4 - Try the egg fast. On the Keto diet you can eat as many eggs as you want. The egg fast is to eat nothing but eggs for one week. There are various ways to cook the eggs to make them pleasant to eat. You can vary the way you cook the eggs so that it does not become boring.

You can boil the eggs or scramble the eggs. With scrambled eggs add some hard shredded cheese. As suggested above It is much better to buy cheese slice or block and grate the cheese yourself.

Suggestion: Break your eggs in a small bowl and

whisk with a fork. Then add the grated cheese and stir it in with the eggs. It gives the eggs a very pleasant taste.

Should you have diabetes, this is a sure way to bring the numbers down. This writer has tested and proven that the egg fast will bring the diabetic numbers down.

Vita-Guard Keto Trick # 5 - Keto Baked Salmon

Ingredients:

- 1 tbsp olive oil

- 2 lbs salmon

- 1 tsp sea salt

- ground black pepper

- 7 oz. butter

- 1 lemon

Instructions

1. Preheat the oven to 400°F

2. Grease a large baking dish with olive oil. Place the salmon, with the skin-side down, in the prepared baking dish. Generously season with salt and pepper.

3. Slice the lemon thinly and place on top of the salmon. Cover with half of the butter in thin slices.

4. Bake on middle rack for about 20–30 minutes, or until the salmon is opaque and flakes easily with a fork.

Heat the rest of the butter in a small sauce pan until it starts to bubble. Remove from heat and let cool a little. Gently add some lemon juice.

Vita-Guard Keto Trick # 5 - Increase your fiber intake.

Just because you're on a Keto diet doesn't mean you should skimp on your fiber intake! One of the struggles with Keto is getting enough fiber.

Most fruits aren't part of a keto diet, and the grains, beans, oatmeal, bread that you used to get fiber from are also out of the question.

That leaves just veggies for most of us...and it's hard to eat enough vegetables and still stay under your net carb requirements. But yet fiber is highly important...

You Need Fiber on Keto - Here's Why:

1. Fiber slows the absorption of glucose and therefore decreases the GI (glycemic index) of a meal.

2. In particular, prebiotic fiber feeds your beneficial or "good" bacteria in your large intestines. These types of fiber pass undigested to your large intestines where they're "eaten" by your gut bacteria. The bacteria in turn produce vitamin B12 and fatty acids that keep your bodies healthy.

Fiber also helps keep our bowel action regular and relieves constipation.

The easiest way to boost your fiber intake is to eat more low carb vegetables, like spinach, kale, broccoli, cauliflower, okra.

Unfortunately, despite most of our best efforts, most of us don't eat even close to enough vegetables. And adding too many vegetables (even low carb ones) can increase your net carbohydrate intake.

The average American eats around 10 grams of fiber per day. And recommended amounts for fiber are over 25 grams per day.

That's why boosting your fiber and veggie intake with a supplement can really help.

Chapter Four

Top Vegetables for Keto Diet

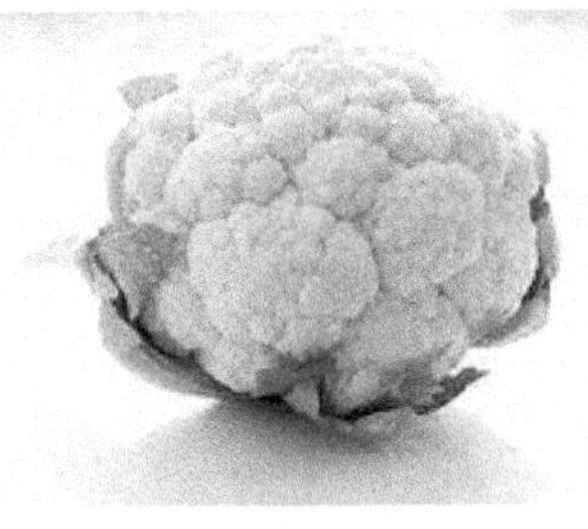

cauliflower

The keto community has gotten particularly creative with cauliflower, using it as a low carb potato substitute and even in place of rice or noodles. If pasta is your downfall, you can use cauliflower as a substitute in dishes like homemade mac and cheese and fettuccini alfredo. If you love those starchy white potatoes, you can make mashed cauliflower dishes to substitute for the high-carb potato dish. You can easily put a keto spin on many of your favorite recipes by simply replacing the high carb ingredient with cauliflower. There are **only 2.9 grams of net carbs** in an entire cup of this popular low carb vegetable, making it a clear winner on a keto diet.

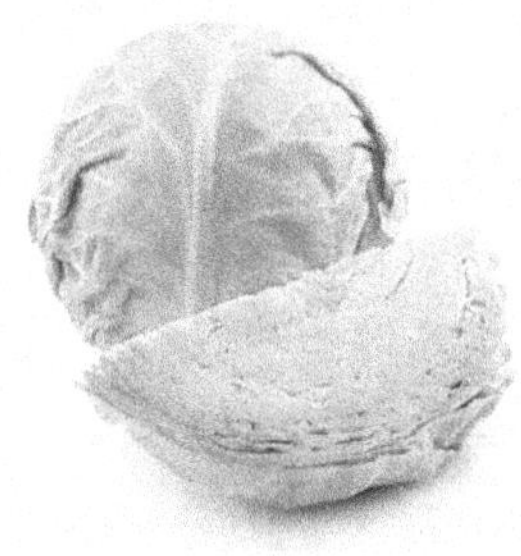

Cabbage

Cabbage contains only **2.3 grams of net carbohydrates** in a single cup, making it a coveted food for anyone on the keto diet. If you are looking for something filling and low in carbs, look no further. You could really chow down before it would have any effect on your state of ketosis. Eaten raw the vegetable can prove a bit bitter, but it can be a tasty addition to many salads. When roasted, cabbage really shines, taking on an almost buttery taste and texture. If cooked in soups or broths, the flavor can be washed out by competing flavors in the dish.

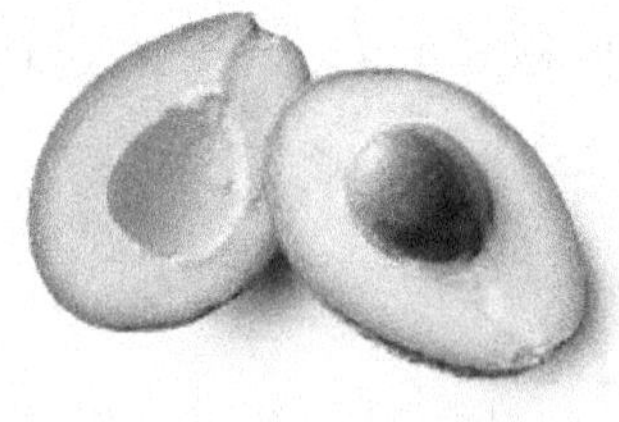

Avocado

Avocado is one of the healthiest low carb veggies (er, fruit actual-ly!) on the planet. Avocado con-tains fiber, copper, folate, and potassium. The fruit also contains Vitamin K, Vitamin E, Vitamin C, and Vitamin B1, B2, B3, B5 and B6. That's a lot of B-Vitamins! It also contains zinc, iron, manganese, and magnesium. With a mere **2 net carbohydrates per 100 grams**, the avocado is a must on the list of acceptable foods on the keto diet. It is low in saturated fats and absent of sodium and cholesterol.

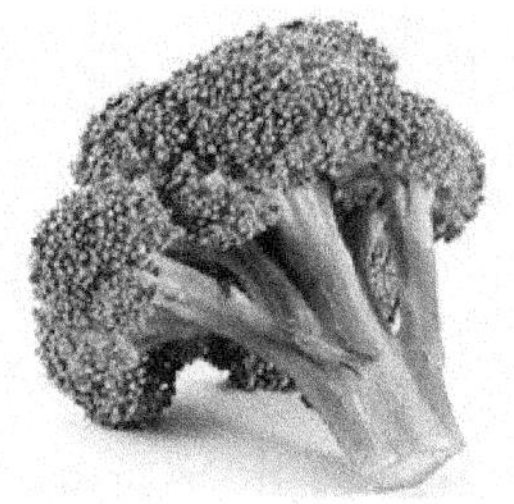

Broccoli

Broccoli is a wonderful vegetable and one of the most popular in the low-carb or keto kitchen. With about 4 percent carbohydrates, it can substitute for rice, pasta and potatoes in a number of ways.

Many people frown upon childhood memories of broccoli boiled into an unrecognizable and bland mush… That's sad because this vegetable can be a vibrantly green source of delight when cooked right – and for this, we recommend our recipes below.

If you've never tried butter-fried broccoli we strongly suggest that you do so, it's absolutely delicious. Or why not make a creamy mash, a filling soup or a flavorful gratin the entire family will love.

One of the things most people struggle with when living the keto lifestyle is sides. We all know we need our veggies, but being on the keto diet means making smart, educated choices even with natural foods like fruits and vegetables.

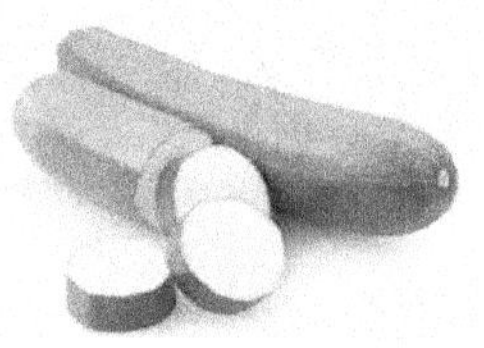

Zucchini

A zucchini (Cucurbita pepo) is a type of summer squash that's rich in nutrition. Though it is botanically thought of as a fruit, it is widely cultivated as a vegetable for domestic consumption in many countries. There are yellow and light green colored varieties. Zucchini contains a wealthy of beneficial micronutrients such as:

- Minerals

- Carotenoids (Plant pigments that have been proven to provide protective health benefits, including reducing cancer risk)

- Vitamin C (58%, important for skin, bones, and connective tissue)

- Other antioxidants that help with anti-carcinogenic, anti-inflammatory, and antimicrobial activities.

One scientific study showed that zucchini could have neuroprotective benefits, meaning that in can help with or result in protecting the nervous systems.

Researchers administered a neurotoxic agent (a cause of brain damage) to sample groups of rats and gave some of the sample rat groups extract of a zucchini peel.

The extract was proven to protect the brain tissue in the rats against brain injuries by restoring antioxidant enzyme activities.

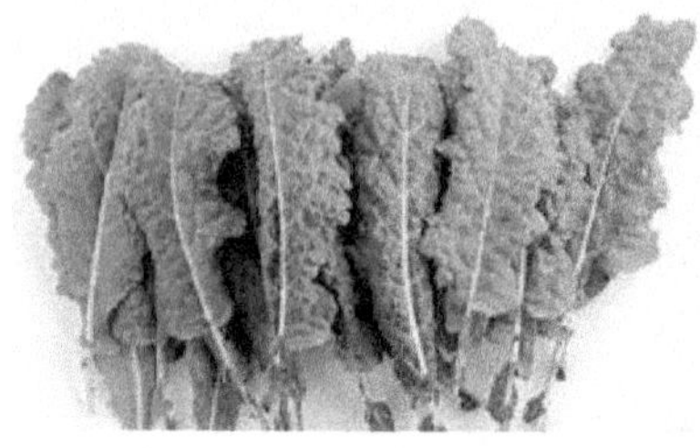

Spinach

When you combine the recommended daily intake of electrolytes with the electrolytes you must supplement on a keto diet, you end up with the following:

- 7300 mg sodium
- 5700 mg potassium
- 700 mg magnesium

In order to meet these requirements, it is generally recommended to take a potassium salt (ex/ nosalt, litesalt, etc) and a magnesium supplement. However, with proper vegetable intake, this is completely unnecessary!

Kale chips, green smoothies, even a good old-fashioned salad, kale seems like it's everywhere these days. And it's easy to under-

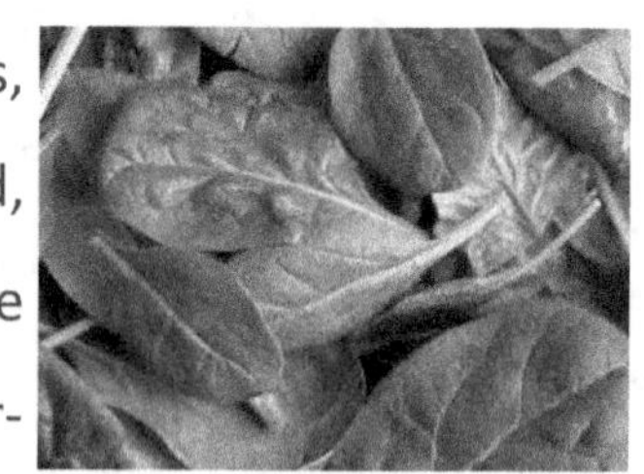

Kale

stand why!

"Kale is jam-packed with vitamins. Eating one cup of chopped kale gets you over 200% of your daily value of vitamin A, 134% of your daily value for vitamin C, and almost 700% of your daily value for vitamin K! In addition, kale contains important minerals like manganese, potassium, and copper." It's a true superfood!

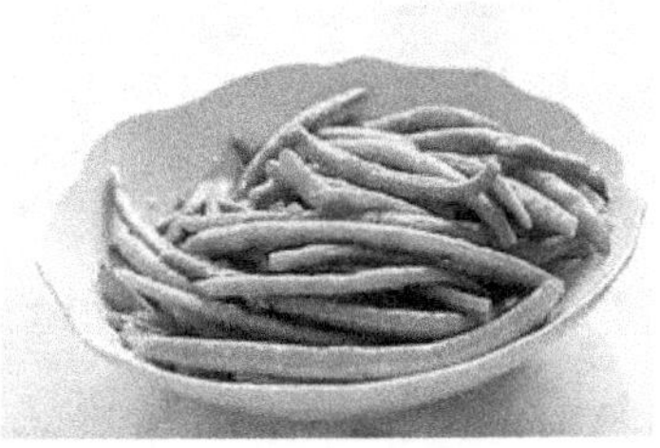
Green Beans

Green beans are a pretty classic side dish in many cultures. They go great with any protein and give a wealth of nutrients. They are also way less dense than their carb-y bean counterparts.

Fresh vs. Frozen

You might be thinking, what about canned? I'm not a big fan of canned vegetables. They contain a lot of extra ingredients (sulfites & sodium) to make them shelf stable for long periods of time. Fresh and frozen vegetables both have their own perks. When it comes to nutrition value, fresh vegetables that are in season will typically always win. Frozen vegetables give you the convenience of sticking a bag in the microwave for a few minutes and having delicious steamed vegetables ready to be devoured.

I highly recommend using fresh green beans because they tend to cook better in the oven. You can buy them trimmed already, or trim them yourself at home easily by just quickly snapping off the little stems.

Bacon Fat

Bacon fat is one of those things that most health nuts would just drain out into the dark abyss and not even give it a second thought. The keto diet consists of eating foods that are high in fat. Thus, I like to use my

bacon fat in recipes if I can. It adds a ton of extra delicious flavor and it's nice to not have anything go to
waste.

Brussels sprouts are also one of the best vegetables for a ketogenic and low carb diet because they are low in carbs and full of fiber. Brussel

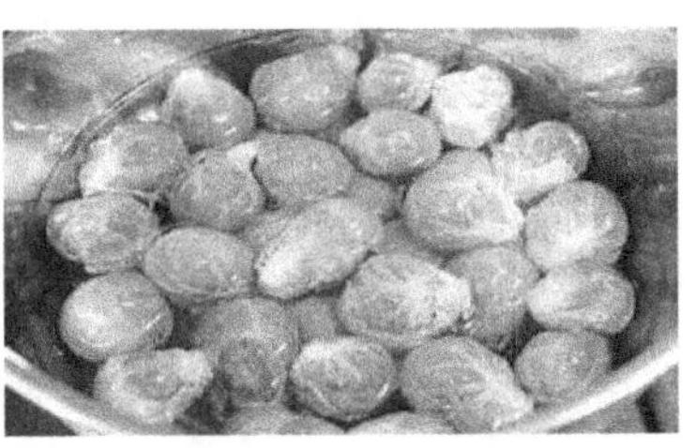

Brussel Sprouts

sprouts are a vegetable that is full of vitamin C and it is a cruciferous vegetable that supports the liver in clearing out toxins such as excessive estrogen which is a risk factor for cancer.

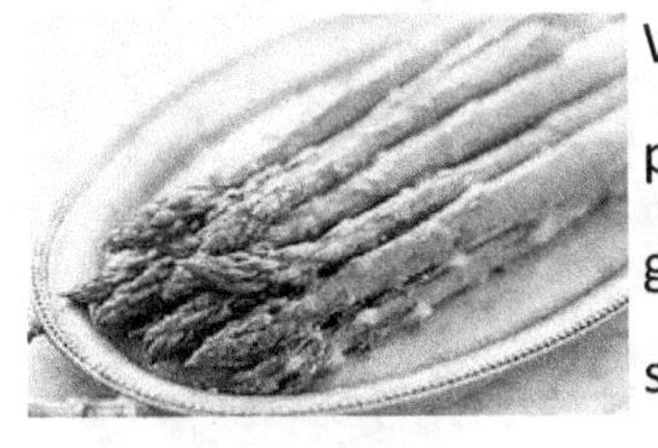

Asparagus

Whether you're a huge fan of as-paragus already or you haven't given the veg much thought, you should be adding more to your plate. Not only does the stalk have several health benefits, but it's also super tasty in salads,

Before and After Pictures of People who lost Weight on the Keto Diet

grain bowls and pasta, or as a roasted side dish. Here's what you get when you eat the green (or white, or purple!) stuff

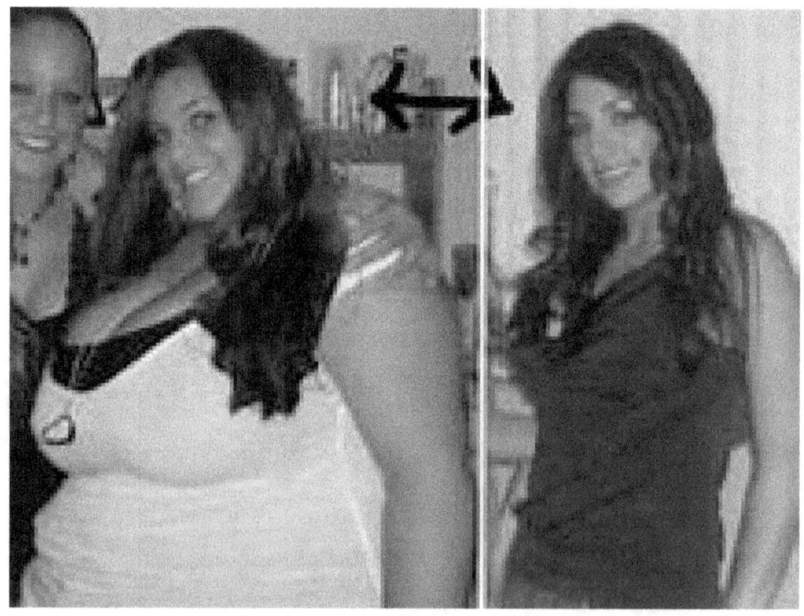

Chapter Five

Best Cooking Oils for Keto

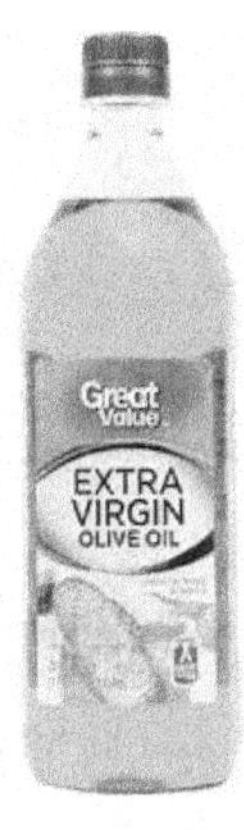

For a diet made up predominantly of fat, you'll want to make sure you stock up on the absolute best cooking oils. That's because the oil you cook with can make or break the perfect meal!

Olive Oil

Take a walk through your grocery store and you'll see shelves stocked with vegetable oils, nut oils, seed oils, olive oils, and more! Not all oils are created equally, though. Some have to go through intense processing before they ever make it to your kitchen. Others have such low smoke points that you may sacrifice their nutritional integrity if you use them to cook over high heat. So what oils are best when cooking for a keto diet?

EXTRA-VIRGIN OLIVE OIL (EVOO). Packed with antioxidants and robust flavor, extra-virgin olive oil is un-refined and minimally processed. Due to its low smoke point, use extra-virgin ol-ive oil for low-heat cooking, dips, and

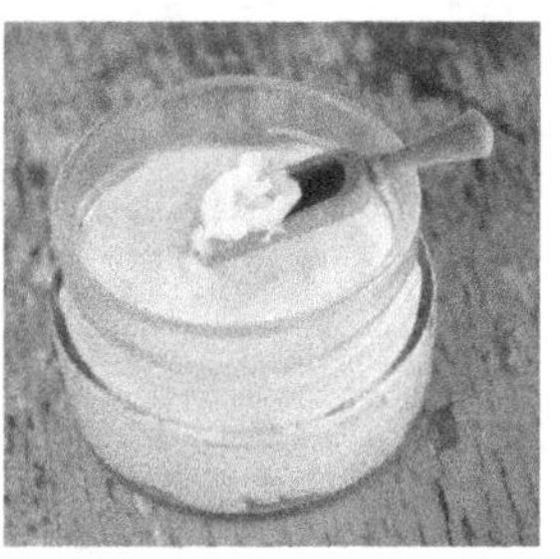

Coconut Oil

dressings. EVOO pairs well with meat, vegetables, and even eggs!

For a recipe utilizing extra Packed with antioxidants and robust flavor, extra-virgin olive oil is unrefined and mini-mally processed. Due to its low smoke point, use extra-virgin olive oil for low-heat cooking, dips, and dressings. EVOO pairs well with meat, vegetables, and even eggs!

For a recipe utilizing EVOO, try this Pancetta and Goat Cheese Stuffed Flank Steak. High in fat, low in carbs, and packed with flavor, it's as delicious as it sounds. Another fan favorite is the Pulled Pork with Cabbage Slaw. It's packed with flavor and easy to make, which makes it an excellent mid-week recipe amidst hectic schedules. If you want to upgrade your salads, give our Kale Salad recipe a go. The vinaigrette combines EVOO with apple cider vinegar and a host of spices for a zesty salad experience. Virgin Olive Oil, try this Pancetta and Goat Cheese Stuffed Flank Steak. High in fat, low in carbs, and packed with flavor, it's as delicious as it sounds. Another fan favorite is the Pulled Pork with Cabbage Slaw. It's packed with flavor and easy to make, which makes it an excellent mid-week recipe amidst hectic schedules. If you want to upgrade your salads, give our Kale Salad recipe a go. The vinaigrette combines EVOO with apple cider vinegar and a host of spices for a zesty salad experience.

If you're struggling to get your healthy fats in on your ketogenic diet, then you shouldn't look much further than coconut oil.

This natural superfood is great for your digestion,

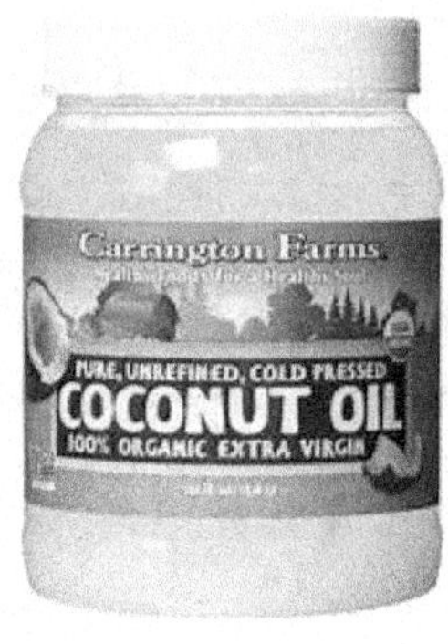

immune system, and can easily be used by the body to provide clean energy from ketones if following a keto diet.

Coconut oil containing MCT oil is one of the simplest types of fat for your body to process well and burn for energy.

Adding it to your high-fat diet is a no brainer.

With a lack of carbs, your body will convert fat into ketones which are used as fuel within the body instead of glucose.

Other than glucose, ketones are the only other source of energy your body can use.

Medium chain triglycerides found in natures coconut oil are efficiently converted into ketones by the body.

MCTs are also useful for those who have difficulty digesting fats.

A little bit of butter goes a long way. Butter is a great source of vitamins A, D, and E, and conjugated linoleic acid (CLA), which has been shown to have anti-cancer properties. It's always preferential to use organic free-range, grass-fed butter as it's generally more nutritionally dense and won't contain any traces of antibiotics.

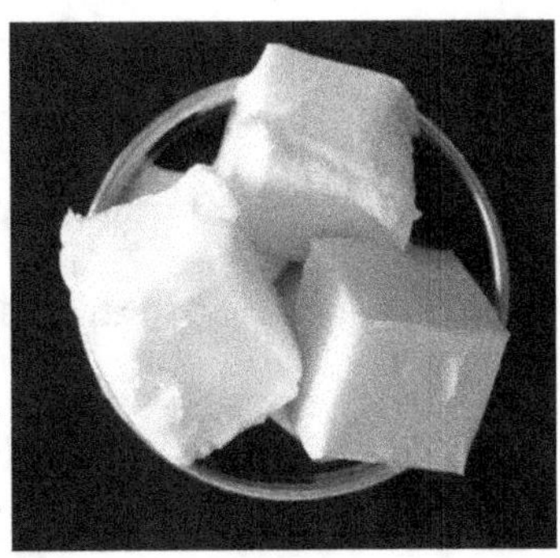

Butter

Regular butter has a low smoke point, so it's best used for cooking under 350 degrees or as a spread. Ghee (clarified butter), on the other hand, has a high smoke point. Try using organic grass-fed ghee for your high-heat cooking needs!

OILS TO AVOID

On the keto diet, you can consume the healthy fats and oils listed above to your heart's desire. However, once again, not all oils are created equal. Oils that go through intense processing — and thus feature processed trans fats — should be avoided at all costs. These types of oils can be damaging to your health for a number of reasons, including increased risk of heart disease, increased risk of cancer, and increased inflammation. As a general rule of thumb, many vegetable and seed oils should be avoided, including:

- Soybean oil
- Canola oil
- Corn oil
- Peanut oil
- Sunflower oil
- Safflower oil
- Cottonseed oil
- Grapeseed oil

You don't have to be afraid of oil or fats when you're on the keto diet. Just make sure you're using the right kinds when you cook.

Before and After Pictures of People who lost Weight on the Keto Diet

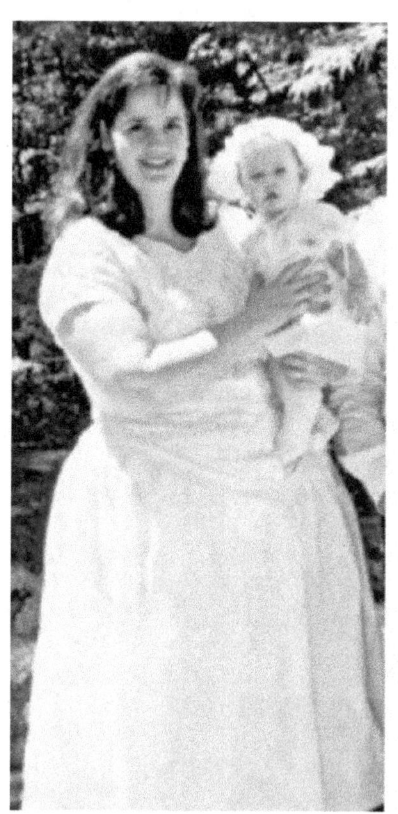 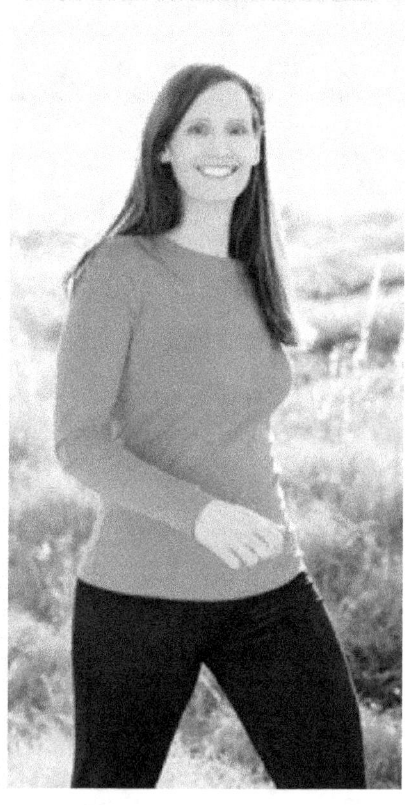

Chapter Six

Low Carb Fruits

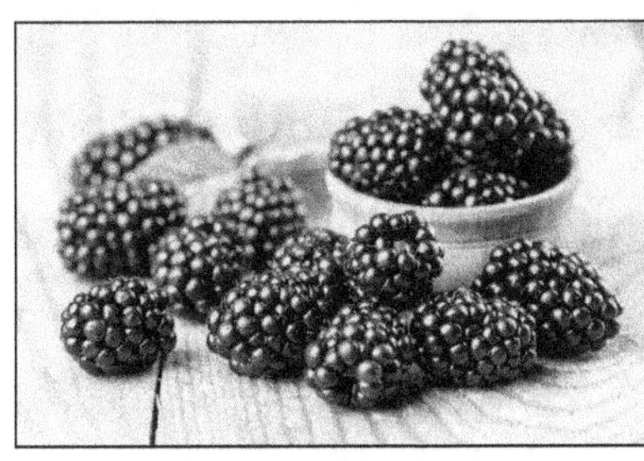

Black Berries

Blackberries have an impressive amount of fiber—nearly two grams in a quarter cup. That serving size also have 1.5 grams of net carbs, so you can definitely add these to your morning yogurt.

Stick with a quarter cup raspberries and you'll get about 1.5 grams of net carbs, per the USDA.

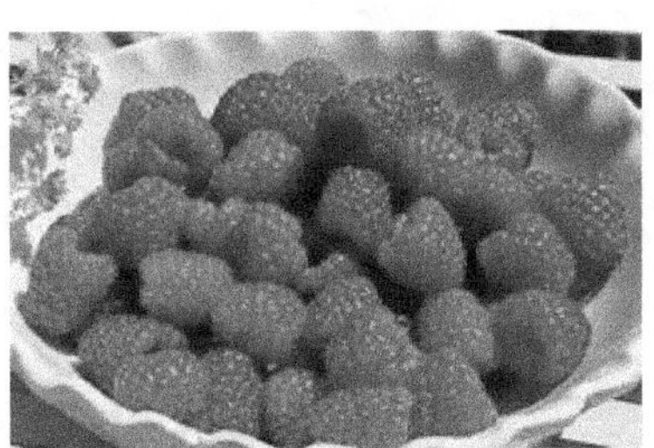

Raspberries

Toss them in a salad, or, even better: whip up heavy whipping cream and toss a few berries on top for a keto-friendly dessert

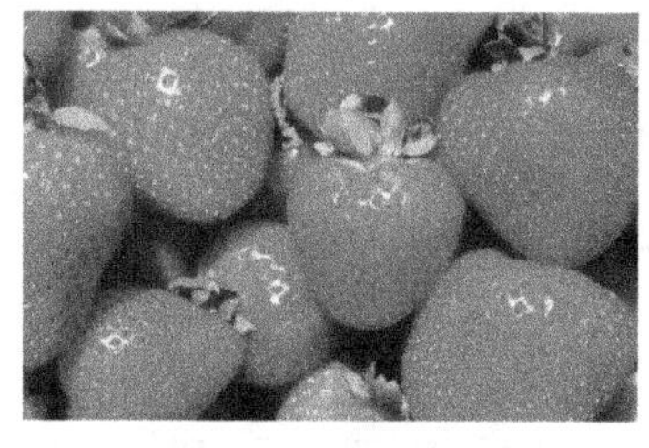

Strawberries

A quarter-cup of strawberry halves contains a little more than two grams of net carbs—or about 10 percent of your daily limit if you're aiming for 20 grams of net carbs a day.

Yet another should-be veggie that's actually a fruit. At two grams of net carbs per half-cup, cherry tomatoes are a great addition to your keto diet.

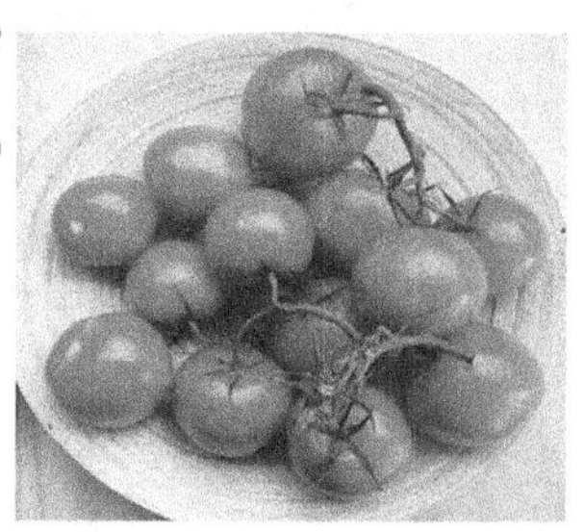

Tomatoes

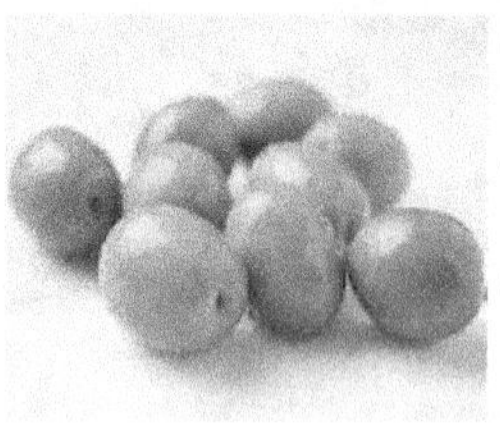

Olives

Olives are another fruit you definitely didn't think were a fruit—so they totally count. Ten small olives pack about three grams of fat and about 1.5 grams of net carbs. Bonus: they're salty, and getting enough sodium is important when following a keto diet

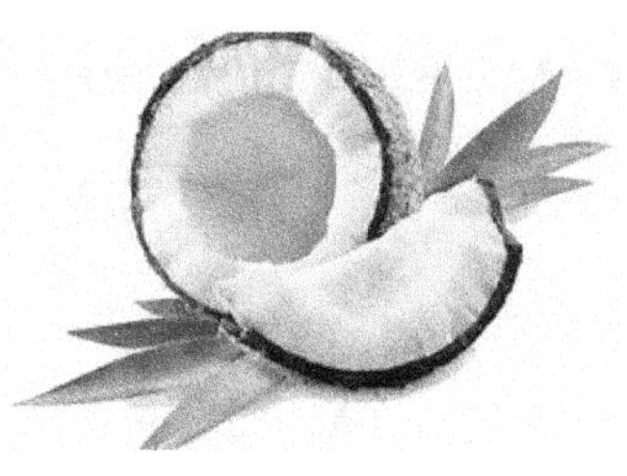

Coconut

One-half cup of shredded coconut meat yields 13 grams of fat, and a respectable 2.5 grams of net carbs. Sugar is often added to coconut, so make sure you're buying unsweetened—or buy an entire coconut and scoop the meat out yourself.

No one's asking you to bite into a lemon—though, if you're into that, you do you—but when you need to dress up unsweetened seltzer water or plain tea, the sour citrus fruit has your back.

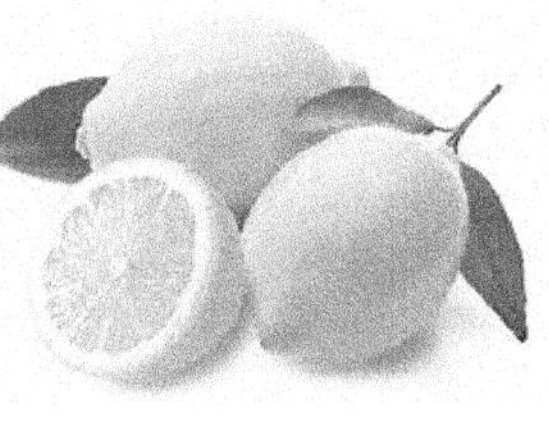

Lemons

A squeeze from a wedge has less than a half of a gram of net carbs. That's a negligible amount of carbs, so honestly, squeeze as many lemons as you want.

There's no denying that the keto diet is all the rage; the high-fat, moderate-protein, super low-carb diet has helped countless people lose impressive amounts of weight. By cutting back so drastically on carbs, the keto diet turns to burning fat for fuel instead of carbs, which puts your body into the fat-burning state of ketosis.

On the keto diet, you should eat 50 grams or fewer of carbs a day. So what does that mean for the foods you can eat? Surprisingly, fruit, which is higher in carbs and fructose than many other natural whole foods, isn't off-limits; you just need to be careful which fruits you decide to eat.

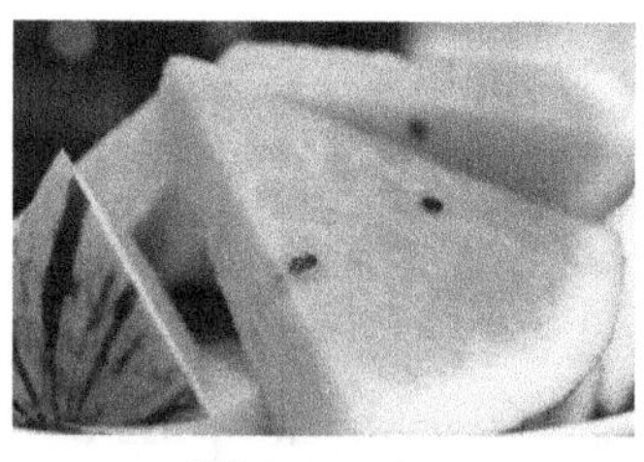

Watermelon

Take watermelon, for example: the delicious Summer treat clocks in at 22 grams of carbs and 18 grams of sugar, with less than two grams of fiber per two-cup serving.

Before and After Pictures of People who lost Weight on the Keto Diet

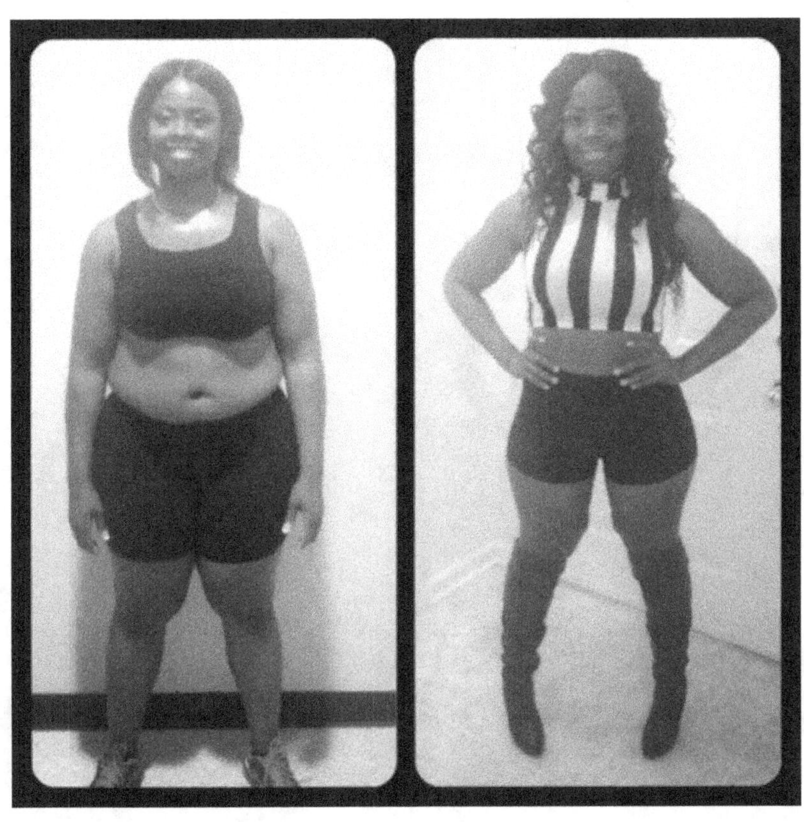

Chapter Seven

Meats for Keto Diet

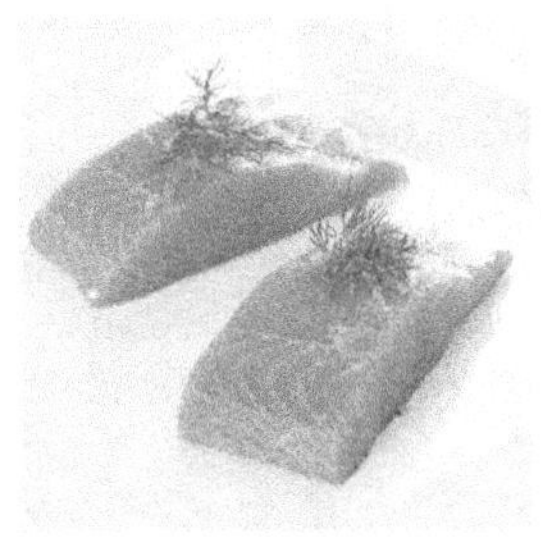

Salmon

Keto Baked Salmon was mentioned earlier, but repeated here for your convenience.

Ingredients:

- 1 tbsp olive oil

- 2 lbs salmon

- 1 tsp sea salt

- ground black pepper

- 7 oz. butter

- 1 lemon

Instructions

1. Preheat the oven to 400°F

2. Grease a large baking dish with olive oil. Place the salmon, with the skin-side down, in the prepared baking dish. Generously season with salt and pepper.

3. Slice the lemon thinly and place on top of the salmon. Cover with half of the butter in thin slices.

4. Bake on middle rack for about 20–30 minutes, or until the salmon is opaque and flakes easily with a fork.

Heat the rest of the butter in a small sauce pan until it starts to bubble. Remove from heat and let cool a little. Gently add some lemon juice.

Salmon is very heavy in fats and will aid your Keto diet tremendously.

The keto diet is all about finding the right balance of macronutrients, or proteins, carbohydrates, and fats. Protein and fats are your friends.

Carbohydrates, on the other hand, will thwart your goals of reaching nutritional ketosis. For most people, the magic number is less than 25g of net carbs a day.

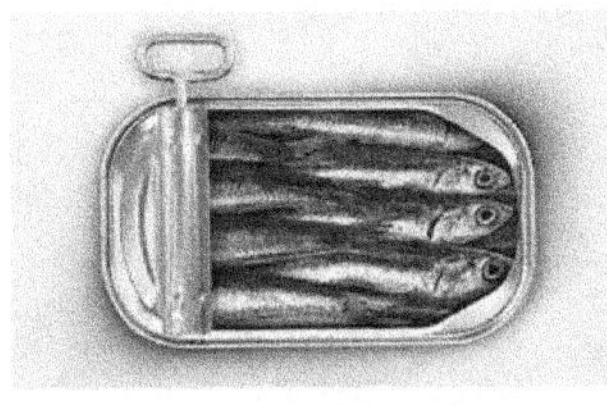

Sardines

And that's where sardines come in. This fish has plenty of protein and fat and negligible carbs. It's a perfect fit with your low-carb keto diet.

In the culinary arts, the word **marbling** refers to white flecks and streaks of fat within the lean sections of meat. Marbling is so named because the streaks of fat resemble a marble pattern. Also called intramuscular fat, marbling adds flavor and is one of the main criteria for judging the quality of cuts of meat. In general, the more marbling it contains, the better a cut of meat is.

Note that we're not talking about the layer of fat on the outside of the steak or roast, which can be trimmed away. Nor are we talking about layers of fat between two separate muscles, like you'll see in chuck roasts, for instance. Marbling is strictly the flecks of fat that occur within the meat itself.

Benefits of Eating Seafood

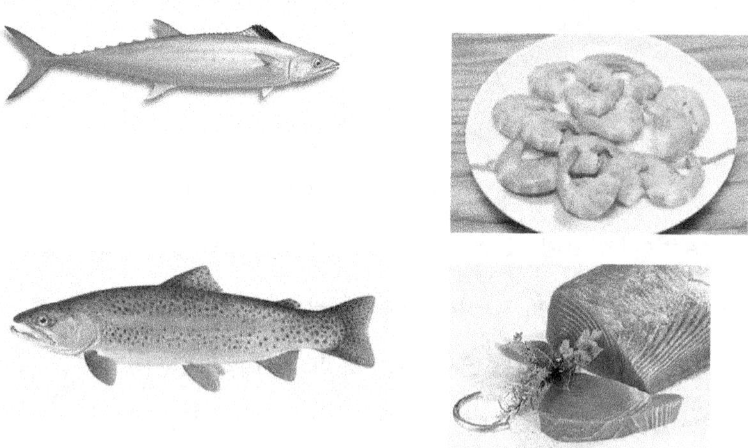

Seafood is extremely rich in a number of nutrients that play an important role in health, and some of them are relatively hard to obtain from other food sources.

It's High in Omega 3 Fatty Acids

Most seafood is high in omega 3 fatty acids, which have a significant impact on your general health, and especially on the health of your cardiovascular system – they lower the risk of heart disease & stroke, help reduce triglycerides levels, lower blood pressure and raise HDL (the "good") cholesterol levels.

Getting sufficient omega 3 from your diet plays a role in mental health – it can help combat depression and anxiety, and can even help with the management of ADHD symptoms in children. It can lower the risk of brain diseases, such as Alzheimer's, and other types of and age-related cognitive deterioration.

Additionally, it lowers inflammation and is beneficial for people suffering from autoimmune diseases, such as psoriasis, arthritis, lupus, Crohn's disease, and more.

Fattier types of fish are considered to be the healthiest out there, exactly because they contain more omega 3 fatty acids.

Which is excellent news for us, ketoers, as on keto you'll likely be consuming more fat than on the standard modern diet, and if you choose the types of fat that are good for you, you'll be aiming for optimal results.

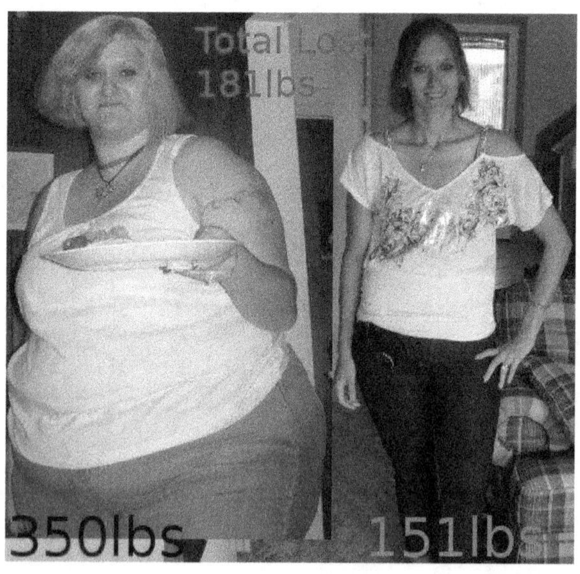

Chapter
Nuts on a Keto Diet

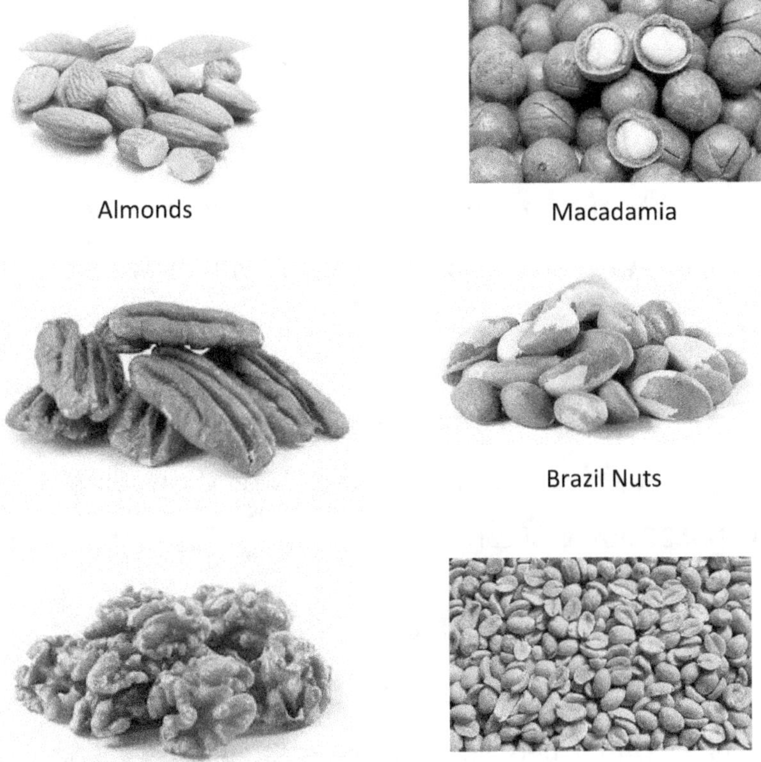

Almonds

Macadamia

Walnuts

Brazil Nuts

Peanuts

Pecans, Brazil nuts and **macadamia nuts**, all on the good side, have the lowest amount of carbs per serving and can be enjoyed freely on the keto diet. At least it's very hard to get too many carbs this way.

Eat these low-carb nuts as a snack (if you need one) between meals, toast and toss into salads and other dishes, or grind them into nut butters to spread into celery, other veggies or low-carb crackers.

The nuts in the middle are not the best keto options, but you can probably get away with a few here and there.

The nuts to the right – especially cashews – should be avoided on keto. You'll very quickly reach the daily keto limit of 20 grams of carbs.

For all these various types of nuts, never eat any version that has been treated with sugar and other glazes, such as with labels like "honey roasted", "sweet chili", "salted caramel" and "spiced." Read labels to make sure that no sugar has been added. These days many brands are adding sugar.

While Brazil, macadamia and pecan nuts are good keto options, you may still want to be a bit restrictive when eating nuts. Especially if you're aiming to lose weight, or reverse type 2 diabetes, even these nuts can still be problematic.

Keep in mind that all nuts contain lots of fat and calories (plus some protein and minerals) – they are very nutritious.

Eating nuts is fine if you're doing so when you're hungry and *need* energy. But if you're just snacking on them between meals – without being hungry – because the nuts taste good or because you're bored, then you're adding tons of fat that you don't need.

The result? Your body will burn the fat from the

nuts, instead of your stored body fat. This is fine if you're happy with your current weight and metabolic health. But if you're aiming to lose weight it's a different story. In that case, reducing snacking between meals to a minimum may be the best option.

Nuts are so tasty and good, that they may be easy to over consume, especially salted varieties.

Adding salt to nuts makes them significantly more rewarding and, for many people, almost addictive.

This can lead to eating far more than you need to feel satiated.

Eating too many nuts, especially with higher carb counts, can seriously slow down weight loss.

Here are some tips to help control consumption, if you need them:

- Select the amount you want to eat.

- **Put the nuts in a small bowl – don't eat out of the full bag or container.**
- Preferably don't mindlessly munch nuts while in front of the TV, watching a movie, reading or doing another activity that has most of your attention
- Aim to instead enjoy them deliberately and mindfully.

Cut back on nuts if you find your weight loss is stalling, and make them an occasional indulgence.

Chapter Seven

Deserts For the keto Diet

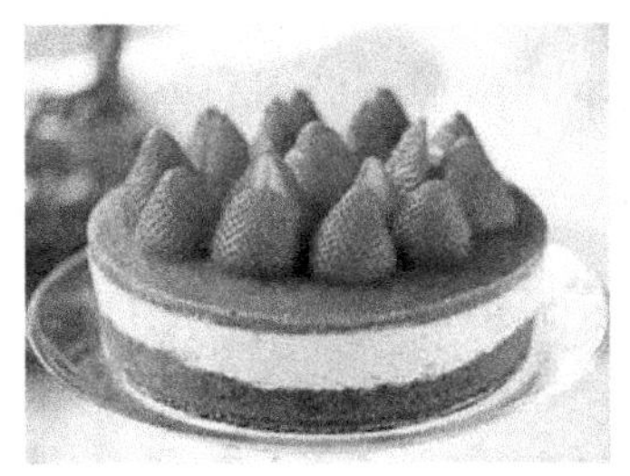
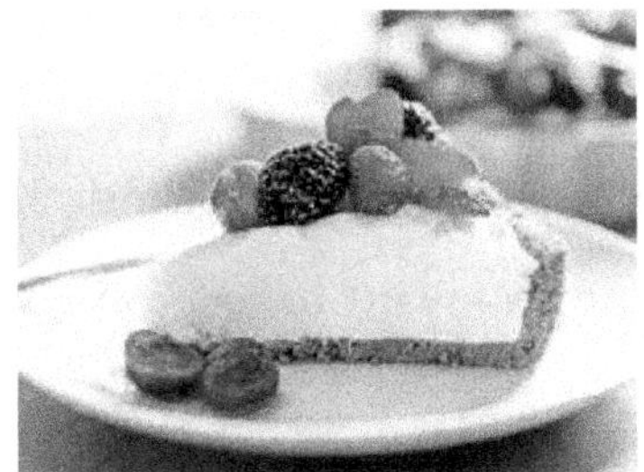

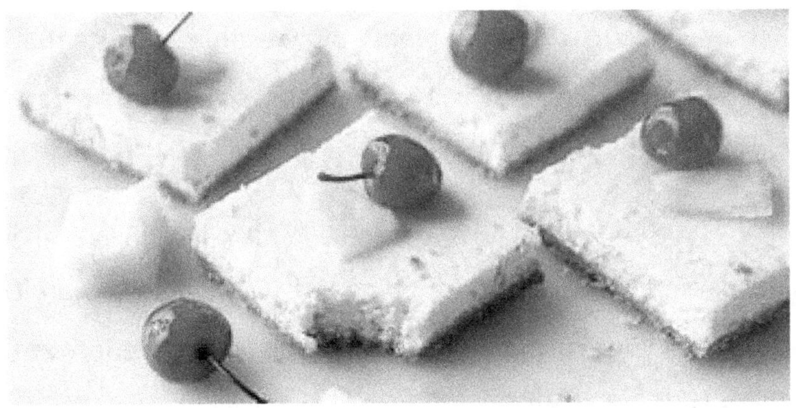

One thing that people really love about the ketogenic diet is that it doesn't make me try to ignore my sweet tooth. Keto desserts are always around to save the day.

When your body enters ketosis, you often find that the craving for sweets disappears.

However, if you've been eating sweet your whole life, like me, then something will mentally trigger you making you want to eat some sweets.

And that's alright!

On keto, there are plenty of awesome desserts that are easy to make that will satisfy your sweet tooth cravings.

You don't have to "eat healthy" by sticking to fruits for dessert. Most fruits are going to be a negative when it comes to your keto diet anyway. The list of keto approved fruits isn't very long.

What's great is that there are so many different keto recipes that you can easily find a substitute for whatever your favorite dessert is and it won't knock you out of ketosis.

Keto baking

Say goodbye to sugar and gluten, say hello to these way healthier low-carb ingredients:

- **Almond flour:** Adds volume, a nutty taste and consistency.

- **Coconut flour:** Tropical taste! Absorbs liquid and is somewhat binding.

- **Ground psyllium husk powder:** Binding agent with a lot of fiber.

- **Full-fat dairy products:** Butter, cream cheese and heavy whipping cream add creaminess, enhance flavor and fullness.

- **Eggs:** Nutritious binding agent.

- **Chocolate:** Preferably sugar-free. The darker the better.

- **Sweeteners:** Some recipes contain natural sweeteners (erythritol and stevia). If you think sweetness from berries, cream, vanilla etc. is enough — skip it.

- **Berries:** Add natural sweetness and color to your dessert.

Part Two

Vita-Guard Keto Products

Details

Different Taste

Not everyone likes certain foods. In the next few pages we want to detail some foods, their values and it is available in tablet or capsule form.

You can enjoy good health without eating the foods you dislike by getting them in capsule form.

You may be surprised at some of the things you read.

Vita-Guard Inflammation Relief

Turmeric Curcumin with Bioperine 1,000 mg

Contains flavonoids, plant-based antioxidants**

Supports overall wellness and a healthy lifestyle**

Capsules can also be opened and prepared as a tea

Contains a one month supply of easy-to-swallow capsules

Turmeric has been used for centuries in Asian cultures for its nutritional properties.** Among the active ingredients in this ancient root are curcuminoids—most notably curcumin—plant-based antioxidants.**

Turmeric contains flavonoids, plant-based antioxidants. Turmeric Curcumin with Bioperine aids in your body's overall well-being.**

** Daily value not established.

Directions: Adults take (1) capsule twice a day preferably with meals.

30 days supply - $36.95

Order from: www.VitaGuardKeto.com

Vita-Guard

Collagen Plus 1,2 & 3

Collagen is a major structural protein in the human body (found in skin, joints, bones, blood vessels and connective tissues.) As we age, collagen naturally breaks down and diminishes over time - leading to the early signs of aging. Vita-Guard Advanced Formula with added Vitamin C is designed to help replenish the body's supply of vital protein.** This product delivers intensive nourishment to help counteract the effects of the aging process.

- Revitalizes skin, hair & nails**

- Fights the effects of aging**

- Replenishes collagen**

- Supports tendons & ligaments**

- Boosts dietary protein**

** No daily values established.

Directions: (Adults) Take (4) tablets per day, all at once or in divided doses.

30 days supply - $39.95

Order from: www.VitaGuardKeto.com

Vita-Guard Healthy Heart

Contains Omega-3, Omega-6 and Omega-9 – the "good" fats important for cellular, heart and metabolic health.**

TRIPLE OMEGA 3-6-9 Fish and Flax Oils contain a proprietary blend of essential oils, including Flaxseed Oil and Ester Omega Fish Oil.

Supports Heart Health.**

Purified to eliminate mercury.

Directions: For adults, take three (2) softgels daily, preferably with a meal.

30 days supply - $28.95

Order from: www.VitaGuardKeto.com

Vita-Guard Keto Burn

Keto Burn was introduced to the panel of invertors on the Shark Tank TV show. They were so impressed that the panel invested $2.5 million. They sold out in the first five minutes. The same product is being offered to through Vita -Guard.

Keto Burn causes small granules to be released in the blood stream. These granules are sometimes called "fat eaters" because they go through the body and eat excessive fat. One customer lost 21 lbs. in two weeks and never changed his eating habits.

Directions: Take (1) caplet twice a day, preferably 30 minutes before meals.

Watch the fat disappear.

30 days supply - $39.95

Order from: www.VitaGuardKeto.com

Vita-Guard Blood Vessel Cleanser

The human body contains 62,000 miles of tiny, blood vessels. The microscopic vessels are so small that x-ray or MRI can not detect them. Since they are so small they get clogged with heavy metals such as chromium, iron, lead, mercury, copper, aluminum, nickel, zinc, calcium, cobalt, manganese, and magnesium , etc.

The only way to cleanse these vessels is with a chelator such as Vita-Guard Blood Vessel Cleanser. This acts as a magnet to bind and flush the blood vessels. It is the only treatment for lead poisoning.

Directions: For adults, take 1 quick release capsule twice a daily, preferably with meals.

30 days supply - $33.95

Order from: www.VitaGuardKeto.com

Vita-Guard Ultra Vitamins

Vita-Guard Ultra vitamins is a rich formula of over 35 ingredients that help in areas of bone maintenance, energy metabolism, immune system support, and antioxidant health.** See Supplement Facts for a complete listing of vitamins and minerals.

Directions: Adults can take (1) Vita-Guard Ultra Vitamin coated tablet in the morning with a meal and (1) Vita-Guard Keto Burn twice a day.

Please see the Vita-Guard Ultra Vitamins complete description on the website (www.VitaGuardKeto.com).

30 days supply - $29.95

Order from: www.VitaGuardKeto.com

Vita-Guard Exotic Herbs

For Men

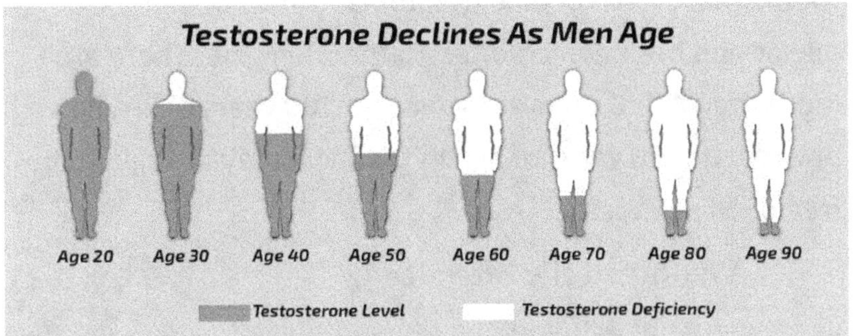

Step 1: Boost Your Free Testosterone Levels Testosterone is central in the male sexual response, including the desire for sex and the mechanics of triggering an erection. High levels of testosterone are associated with a strong desire for sex and an increased ability to have an erection.[1,2]

Step 2: Increase Blood Flow To Your Penis A better blood flow means that the cavities in your penis will fill up with blood more readily. This counters the effects of weak erections. You gain the power to have an erection on demand, maintain it for longer and experience better sex.*

Step 3: Improve Your Libido & Sexual Stamina There are some ingredients that will improve the mood and desire for sex. These have long been known as aphrodisiacs in traditional Chinese medicine, products that include these ingredients may increase your sex drive and libido which does drop in men at a certain age.*

Directions: For Adult Men, take two (2) capsules daily, preferably with a meal.

30 days supply - $32.95 Order from: www.VitaGuardKeto.com

Life Extender

The Vita-Guard Life Entender is the whole cordyceps mush-room. These have been eaten for centuries by the Oki-nawas and has been credited to their long life. There are more than 400 Okinawas living past 100 years old. When one reaches 90 years of age in Okinawa they are said to be free of all diseases.

Vita-Guard Life Extender

- Manages Type II Diabetes
- Can Treat Liver Diseases
- Can Treat Kidney Diseases
- Has Anti-Aging Properties
- May Be Effective Against Tumors
- May Increase Longevity
- Has Many Fertility Benefits
- Helping to Combat Fatigue
- May help treat Crohn's Disease
- Boosting the Immune System
- May Boost Exercise Performance

30 Days supply. $33.95

Order from VitaGuardKeto.com

Anti-Cancer

Anti-inflammatory properties, Manages Type II Diabetes, May help to prevent ulcers, May help to lower blood pressure, May help to treat herpes, May help to prevent or treat cancer, Has Anti-Aging Properties, May Be Effective Against Tumors, May Increase Longevity, May help treat Crohn's Disease.

Supplement Facts

Serving Size 2 Capsules. Amount Per Serving % Daily Value Graviola (leaf) 1300 mg*, *Daily Value not established.

Directions: For adults, take two (2) capsules daily, preferably with meals.

These dosages have not been approved by the United States Food and Drug Administration (FDA).

This product is not intended for pregnant or nursing mothers or children under the age of 18, or persons with a known medical condition including any cardiovascular disorder and hypotension (low blood pressure).

60 Capsules. $25.95

Order from: VitaGuardKeto.com

Teen Gold

Directions: Directions: As a dietary supplement, take two (2) jellies per day. Chew thoroughly before swallowing. It's tough out there, stay a step ahead by keeping healthy. Yum -V's complete multivitamin makes it easy for teens to get 15 essential vitamins and minerals, including 100% of the daily requirement of Vitamin C and 800 IU of vitamin D. Yum-V's complete multivitamin for teens also contains 1000 mcg of Biotin which helps support healthy skin, nails, and hair to help you look your best.

Supplement Facts

Serving Size: 2 Jellies, Servings Per Bottle: 30

Amount Per Serving % Daily Value . Calories 15

Total Carbohydrates 4 g 1% , Sugars 4 g **

Vitamin A (as all trans retinyl acetate) 2200 IU 44%

Vitamin C (as ascorbic acid) 60 mg 100%

Vitamin D (as Cholecalciferol) 800 IU 200%

Vitamin E (as DL-alpha tocopheryl acetate) 15 IU 50%

Niacin (as Niacinamide) 12 mg 60%

Vitamin B6 (as pyridoxine HCl) 4 mg 200%

Folate (as folic acid) 400 mcg 100%

Vitamin B12 (as cyanocobalmine) 12 mcg 200%

Biotin 1000 mcg 333%

Pantothenic Acid (as calcium pantothenate) 10 mg 100%

Iodine (as potassium iodide) 40 mcg 26%

Zinc (as zinc citrate) 1 mg 6%, Sodium 10mg <1%

Choline (as choline chloride) 60 mcg ** . Inositol 40 mcg **

†Percent Daily Values are based on a 2,000 calorie diet

**Daily Value not established

60 Jellies $27.95

Order from VitaGuardKeto.com

Energy Tonic

About Energy Tonic

Each of these ingredients separately have hundreds of health benefits. Together they are amazingly powerful to provide the best formulation that one can consume.

Ingredients:

Raw honey, Lemon juice from concentrate, Apple cider vinegar. Purified water. Ingredients carefully formulated with low heat.

Supplement Facts

Serving size 1 Oz. Serving per container 16. Amount per serving % DV

Calories .05**. Sugar 2.8**

Folate 0.75**. It contains virtually no fiber, fat or protein .

2-16 oz. Bottles $12.95

Order from VitaGuardKeto.com

Avocado Oil Capsules

One of the World's Most Nutritious Foods

Promotes healthy cholesterol and triglyceride levels. Avocado oil is rich in oleic acid, an omega-9 essential fatty acid.

Supports healthy skin, joints and connective tissues.

Organic.

Supplement Facts

Serving Size 1 Softgel **Amount Per Serving % Daily Value** Calories 10 Total Fat 1g 1% Certified Organic Virgin Avocado Oil 1 g * (Persea gratissima) (fruit): Typical Fatty Acid Profile: Omega-6—Linoleic Acid 6-16% Omega-9—Oleic Acid 54-74%

Percent Daily Values are based on a 2,000 calorie diet.

*Daily Value not established.

60 Softgels $27.95

Order from VitaGuardKeto.com

Blueberry Eye Bright
Healthy Eyesight

Provides powerful antioxidant support for every cell in your body, including the eye's cells**Blueberry extract is a natural source of two important phytochemicals, anthocyanins and chlorogenic acid, to support antioxidant health**Eyebright provide additional herbal support for good health Marigold and Grape Seed extracts are included for extra nutritional support. Our vegetarian-friendly caplets are coated for ease of swallowing.

Supplement Facts

Serving Size 2 Caplets **Servings Per Container 60 Amount Per Serving% Daily Value** Blueberry 2,000 mg (2.0 g) ** (Vaccinium spp.)Vaccinium myrtillus) (fruit) (From 400 mg of a 5:1 Extract) Eyebright 1,000 mg (1.0 g) ** (Euphrasia officinalis) (aerial) (From 200 mg of a 5:1 Extract)Marigold 400 mg ** (Tagetes erecta) (flower) (From 80 mg of a 5:1 Extract) Grape Seed 200 mg ** (Vitis vinifera) (seed) (From 40 mg of a 5:1 Extract) ***Daily Value not established.

Directions: For adults, take two (2) caplets daily, preferably with a meal. **Other Ingredients:** Dextrose, Dicalcium Phosphate, Vegetable Cellulose. Contains <2% of: Silica, Vegetable Magnesium Stearate, Vegetable Stearic Acid. No Artificial Color, Flavor or Sweetener, No Preservatives, No Milk, No Lactose, No Soy, No Gluten, No Wheat, No Yeast, No Fish. Sodium Free.

 120 Caplets

Order from: VitaGuardKeto.com

Celery Seed Capsules

Celery seed is derived from the common kitchen staple, celery. The seeds of this vegetable have been used for centuries in Ayurvedic wellness traditions. Our celery seed quick-release capsules deliver the equivalent of 1000 mg to your body per serving! Instead of cooking up celery, take these convenient capsules for countless benefits!

Supplement Facts

Serving Size: 1 Quick Release Capsule. **Servings Per Container:** 240 **Amount Per Serving% Daily Value (DV)** Celery Seed (Apium graveolens) (from 250 mg of 4:1 Extract)1,000 mg*

Other ingredients: Rice Powder, Gelatin Capsule, Vegetable Magnesium Stearate

Directions: For adults, take 1 quick release capsule 1 to 3 times daily, preferably with meals.

240 Capsules

Order from: VitaGuardKeto.com

Kale Capsules

One of the World's Healthiest Foods

A leafy vegetable, kale has been used across cultures and cuisines for centuries. Kale refers to a specific variety of vegetable closely related to cabbage, broccoli and sprouts. Used for centuries, with its ancestors use documented as far back as the ancient Greeks and Romans, kale was a popularly cultivated green vegetable throughout the Middle Ages. Its cultivation was encouraged during World War II during war time rationing to help supplement important nutrients that otherwise may have been lacking from daily diets. Kale is known for its rich nutritional profile and its ability to be cultivated in the winter, which has made it a popular ingredient in many dishes.

Vita-Guard Kale Supplement Pills (800mg) are available in easy-to-swallow quick release capsules for easy absorption that are ideal for those that want to experience its nutritional benefits of kale but do not enjoy the taste of the vegetable.

Supplement Facts

Serving Size: 1 Quick Release Capsule

Servings Per Container: 60

Amount

Per Serving% Daily Value

(DV) Kale (Brassica oleracea) (leaf) (from 200 mg of 4:1 extract)800 mg***Other ingredients:** Rice Powder, Gelatin Capsule, Vegetable Magnesium Stearate, Silica

Directions: For adults, take 1 quick release capsule daily, preferably with a meal.

WARNING: If you are pregnant, nursing, taking any medications or have any medical condition, consult your doctor before use. If any adverse reactions occur, immediately stop using this product and consult your doctor. If seal under cap is damaged or missing, do not use. Keep out of reach of children. Store in a cool, dry place. **Other Information:** Equivalent from 200 mg of 4:1 extract.* Daily Value (DV) not established.

60 Capsules $27.95

Order from: VitaGuardKeto.com

Sea Cucumber Capsules

Introducing the deep sea nutrition of Vita-Guard Sea Cucumber! Used for centuries in China as a valuable source of nourishment for joint health, sea cucumber is rich in chondroitin sulfate and other important nutrients for joint tissue maintenance.

Sea cucumbers are very low in calories and fat and high in protein, making them a weight loss-friendly food. They also contain many powerful substances, including antioxidants, which are **good** for your health. **Sea cucumbers** are high in protein, with most species consisting of 41–63% protein (4, 5).

100 Capsules $33.95

Order from: VitaGuardKeto.com

Olive Oil Capsules

Our Olive Leaf Extract is derived from the leaves of the Mediterranean olive tree. This extract is standardized for 20% Oleuropein, a powerful phytonutrient. Olive leaves have been used for overall well-being for thousands of years by people in countries bordering the Mediterranean.

Supplement Facts

Serving Size 1 capsule

Amount Per Serving% Daily Value Olive Leaf Extract 150 mg ** (Olea europaea) (standardized to contain 20% Oleuropein, 30 mg)**Daily Value not estab-lished.**Directions:** For adults, take one (1) capsule up to three times daily, preferably with meals. Capsules may be opened and prepared as a tea.

Other Ingredients: Vegetable Cellulose, Gelatin. Contains <2% of: Silica, Vegetable Magnesium Stearate.

WARNING: If you are pregnant, nursing, taking any medications or have any medical condition, consult your doctor before use. Discontinue use and consult your doctor if any adverse reactions occur. Not intended for use by persons under the age of 18. Keep out of reach of children. Store at room temperature. Do not use if seal under cap is broken or missing.

No Artificial Color, Flavor or Sweetener, No Preservatives, No Sugar, No Starch, No Milk, No Lactose, No Soy, No Gluten, No Wheat, No Yeast, No Fish, Sodium Free.

60 Capsules $33.95

Order from: VitaGuardKeto.com

Vita-Guard Super Food

About the product

- SUPERCHARGE YOUR METABOLISM & ENERGY LEVELS from week 1- Give your body the best raw materials to create the most energy NATURALLY SO you will feel more ENERGETIC and RESTED

- BOOST YOUR MEMORY AND FOCUS, Vita-Guard Capsules are the top Premium Superfood Containing Essential Vitamins & Minerals, 46 Antioxidants, 35 Anti-inflammatory, All 9 Essential Amino Acids.

- PROMOTE GOOD MOOD, Contains high amounts of the vitamins A, B, C, and E and the minerals potassium, iron and calcium and a number of antioxidants. The vitamin content of this food can help to treat depression that is caused by a nutrient deficiency. A vitamin imbalance can lead to hormonal imbalances and sleep pattern disturbances that cause or increase depression in some cases.

- THE 'MIRACLE TREE' -Our 100% NATURAL Moringa is

exactly what your body needs as it transitions. You'll get a super dosage of nutrients to boost your energy and mood as you drop the weight! Our Premium Moringa is your ticket to a whole new you!

Moringa oleifera trees are grown mostly in Central Asia.

9 times more protein than yogurt

15 times more potassium than bananas

17 times more Calcium than milk

7 times more vitamin C than oranges

9 times more vitamin A than carrots

25 times more iron than spinach

92 nutrients

46 antioxidants

Omega 3, 6, & 9

Vitamins A to Z

Directions: Take 2 capsule each day with food and a glass of water.

90 Capsules $45.95

Order from: VitaGuardKeto.com

Spinach Capsules

Want to be strong to the finish, but just don't like spinach? New Swanson Premium Brand Full-Spectrum Spinach capsules deliver all the green goodness without the bitter flavor. While they can't replace a healthy diet including the goodness of leafy greens, they can help make up the difference when you just can't bring yourself to eat like everyone's favorite cartoon sailor.

- Full-spectrum spinach capsules feature beneficial thykaloids, chlorophyll and more
- All the green goodness without the bitter flavor
- 400 mg of spinach per single-capsule serving

Serving Information

- Serving Size: 1 capsule
- 400 mg Per Serving
- 90 Servings Per Container $26.95

Order from: VitaGuardKeto.com

Artichoke Capsules

Artichokes, the heart-shaped green vegetables, offer a whole host of nutritional benefits. Grown originally in Southern Europe, the artichoke is one of the oldest health-promoting plants used in folk wellness traditions. You can start enjoying some of its benefits today with our Artichoke Leaves supplement that delivers the equivalent of 520 mg to your body in quick-release capsules!

Additional Information:

Artichokes, the heart-shaped green vegetables, offer a whole host of nutritional benefits. Grown originally in Southern Europe, the artichoke is one of the oldest health-promoting plants used in folk wellness traditions. You can start enjoying some of its benefits today with our Artichoke Leaves supplement that delivers the equivalent of 520 mg to your body in quick-release capsules!

No Gluten, Non-GMO, No Soy, No Artificial Color, No Artificial Flavor, No Artificial Sweetener, No Preservatives, No Wheat, No Yeast, No Milk, No Lactose

Supplement Facts

Serving Size: 1 Quick Release Capsule

Servings Per Container: 90 **Amount**

Per Serving% Daily Value (DV) Artichoke (Cynara scolymus) (leaf) (from 130 mg of 4:1 extract)520 mg***Other ingredients:** Rice Powder, Gelatin Capsule, Vegetable Magnesium Stearate.

Directions: For adults, take 1 quick release capsule daily, preferably with a meal.

WARNING: If you are pregnant, nursing, taking any medications or have any medical condition, consult your doctor before use. Avoid this product if you are allergic to ragweed or daisy-like flowers. If any adverse reactions occur, immediately stop using this product and consult your doctor. Not intended for use by persons under the age of 18. If seal under cap is damaged or missing, do not use. Keep out of reach of children. Store in a cool, dry place.

Other Information: Equivalent from 130 mg of 4:1 Extract* Daily Value (DV) not established.

90 Capsules $25.95

Order from: VitaGuardKeto.com

Cayenne Capsaicin Capsule

Ultra Max Cayenne Plus is Piping Rock's bona fide super-supplement for peak circulatory health!** Sourced from superior-quality natural ingredients, this Cayenne supplement is packed with cayenne extract, ginger root and hawthorn berry to promote robust, free flowing circulation.** It may also help maintain blood cholesterol levels that are already in the normal range.** Combining three time-tested herbs in one powerful supplement, Piping Rock Ultra Max Cayenne Plus is your ultimate support formula for blood health, circulatory health and cardiovascular well-being!**

Supplement Facts

Serving Size: 2 Quick Release Capsules

Servings Per Container: 50

Cayenne Pepper (Capsicum annuum) (fruit) (40,000 heating units) 450 mg

Ginger (Zingiber officinale) (root) 210 mg **
Hawthorn (Crataegus laevigata) (berry) 210 mg **
Other ingredients: Gelatin Capsule, Rice Powder, Vegetable Magnesium Stearate .

Directions: For adults, take 2 quick release capsules daily, preferably with a meal.

WARNING: If you are pregnant, nursing, taking any medications or have any medical condition, consult your doctor before use. If any adverse reactions occur, immediately stop using this product and consult your doctor. If seal under cap is damaged or missing, do not use. Keep out of reach of children. Store in a cool, dry place.

- Daily Value (DV) not established.

100 Capsules $27.95

Order from: VitaGuardKeto.com

Triple Mushroom Complex

Reishi mushrooms are used in traditional Chinese health practices, and have been used in China for their healthy properties for at least 2,000 years.

Maitake has also been used traditionally for its healthy properties. It contains the beneficial polysaccharide compound, Beta Glucan.

Supplement Facts

Serving Size 1 Capsule

Amount Per Serving% Daily Value

Organic Red Reishi Mushroom Extract 100 mg

* (Ganoderma lucidum) (fruiting body)Organic Shiitake Mushroom Extract 100 mg * (Lentinula edodes) (fruiting body)Organic Maitake Mushroom Extract 100 mg

* (Grifola frondosa) (fruiting body) (a 4:1 Extract, equivalent to 400 mg of Maitake Mushroom)Organic Red Reishi Mushroom Extract30 mg * (Ganoderma lucidum) (fruiting body) (Standardized to contain 4% Triterpenes and 12.5% Polysaccharides)Shiitake Mushroom Extract1.5 mg

* (Lentinula edodes) (fruiting body) (a 20:1 Extract, equivalent to 30 mg of Shiitake Mushroom)*

Daily Value not established.

Directions: For adults, take one (1) capsule once or twice daily, preferably with meals.

Other Ingredients: Vegetable Cellulose, Vegetable Magnesium Stearate.

WARNING: If you are pregnant, nursing, taking any medications or have any medical condition, consult your doctor before use. Discontinue use and consult your doctor if any adverse reactions occur. Keep out of reach of children. Store at room temperature. Do not use if seal under cap is broken or missing.

60 Capsules $27.95

Order from VitaGuardKeto.com

Garlic & Ginger Capsules

This product contains the harmonious combination of garlic and ginger. Garlic contains the original amino acids, vitamins and minerals, including selenium, and special sulphur compounds, including alliin, alliinase, allicin and diallyl disulfide compounds, naturally occurring in garlic. Ginger is naturally dried and not subjected to any additional heat.

Supplement Facts

Serving Size 1 Capsule
Servings Per Container 100
Amount per Serving %DV Odor Modified Garlic (Allium sativum) 500 mg † Organic Ginger Root (4:1 concentrate) (Zingiber Officinale) 200 mg ††Daily Value not established.

Directions: Take 1 capsule 1 to 2 times per day with meals or as directed by your qualified healthcare professional.
Other Ingredients: Magnesium stearate (vegetable source) and silicon dioxide. Capsule consists of gelatin.
WARNING: Keep out of reach of children

100 Capsules $28.95

Order from: VitaGuardKeto.com

Vita-Guard Lemon Balm
Natural Calm & Sleep

For over 2,000 years, lemon balm has been used to calm the mind and take the edge off daily stress.** Planetary Herbals Lemon Balm Full Spectrum™ contains the full range of compounds that occur in the plant naturally. Lemon Balm Full Spectrum is ideal for the temporary relief of normal everyday stress, occasional anxiety, and for promoting a calm, positive mood.**

Supplement Facts

Serving Size: 2 Capsules

Amount Per Serving% Daily Value

Lemon Balm Aerial Parts 1 g

Directions: 2 capsules daily

Other Ingredients: gelatin (capsule), acacia gum, and magnesium stearate.

WARNING: If you are pregnant, may become pregnant, or breastfeeding, consult your health care professional before using this product. Do not use if either tamper-evident seal is broken or missing. Keep out of the reach of children. Store in a cool, dry place.

120 Capsules $39.95

Order from VitaGuardKeto.com

Beet Root Capsules

- Overview. The **beet** is a bulbous, sweet root vegetable that most people either love or hate. ...
- Helps lower blood pressure. ...
- Improves exercise stamina. ...
- May improve muscle power in people with heart failure. ...
- May slow the progression of dementia. ...
- Helps you maintain a healthy weight. ...
- May prevent cancer. ...
- Good source of potassium.

No Gluten, Non-GMO, No Soy, No Artificial Color, No Artificial Flavor, No Artificial Sweetener, No Preservatives, No Wheat, No Yeast, No Milk, No Lactose.

Supplement Facts

Serving Size: 2 Quick Release Capsules**Servings Per Container:** 60 **Amount**

Per Serving% Daily Value

(DV) Beet Root (Beta vulgaris)1,000 mg*

Other ingredients: Rice Powder, Gelatin Capsule, Vegetable Magnesium Stearate, Silica

Directions: For adults, take 2 quick release capsules up to 3 times daily, preferably with meals.

WARNING: If you are pregnant, nursing, taking any medications or have any medical condition, consult your doctor before use. If any adverse reactions occur, immediately stop using this product and consult your doctor. If seal under cap is damaged or missing, do not use. Keep out of reach of children. Store in a cool, dry place.* Daily Value (DV) not established.

120 Capsules $27.95

Order from: VitaGuardKeto.com

Broccoli Sprout Extract

Broccoli Sprout Extract 1000 mg. supports a healthy immune system and healthy cell replication. A number of studies have shown that a diet rich in cruciferous vegetables such as broccoli, Brussels sprouts, cabbage and cauliflower can be beneficial to your health. Researchers have isolated a key component of broccoli called sulforaphane, which may have many protective properties. Sulforaphane, an isothiocyanate, is believed to stimulate enzymes in the body. Freshly germinated broccoli sprouts contain from 30 to 50 times the concentration of isothiocyanates as mature broccoli.

Broccoli Sprout Extract 1000 mg. Benefits:

- Supports healthy immune system
- Supports healthy cell replication
- Supports phase 2 detoxification
- GMP certified
- No artificial colors, flavors, sweeteners or preservatives

As a dietary supplement, take two (2) capsules daily with food, or as directed by your qualified healthcare professional.

Ingredients

**Best Naturals - Broccoli Sprout Extract 1000 mg.
120 Capsules**
Supplement Facts **Serving Size: 2 Capsules Servings Per Container: 60 Amount Per Serving% Daily Value**
Broccoli Sprout (Brassica Oleracea) (Standardized to 6% glucosinolates and 0.3% Sulforaphane) (sprouts)1,000 mg** Daily Value not established.

Other Ingredients: Gelatin, Silica, Vegetable Stearate.

120 Capsules $39.95

Order from: VitaGuardKeto.com

Children's Vita-Bites

Vita-Guard Vita-Bites is the great tasting children's chewable multivitamin made with natural flavors. This delicious orange-flavored tablet provides active, growing children with ten essential vitamins for proper growth and development. Mothers will love vitamin-time because their children do! Preservative Free!

Supplement Facts

Serving Size 1/2 Wafer for Children 2-4 Years of Age; 1 Wafer for Children 4 and Up

Servings Per Container 100; 200 Total Carbohydrate **<1 g <1%*Sugars **<1 g ** Vitamin A (as Retinyl Acetate) 1,250 IU 50% 2,500 IU 50% Vitamin C (as Ascorbic Acid) 30 mg 75% 60 mg 100% Vitamin D (as Cholecalciferol) 200 IU 50% 400 IU 100%Vitamin E7.5 IU 75% 15 IU 50% (as d-Alpha Tocopheryl Acetate)Thiamin0.52 mg 74% 1.05 mg 70% (Vitamin B-1) (as Thiamin Mononitrate) Riboflavin (Vitamin B-2) 0.6 mg 75% 1.2 mg 71% Niacin (as Niacinamide) 6.75 mg 75% 13.5 mg 68%Vitamin B-60.52 mg 74% 1.05 mg 53% (as Pyridoxine Hydrochloride) Folic Acid150 mcg 75% 300 mcg 75%Vitamin B-122.25 mcg 75% 4.5 mcg

75% (as Cyanocobalamin) *Percent Daily Values are based on a 2,000 calorie diet.**Daily Value not established.**Directions:** For adults and children 4 years of age and over, chew one (1) wafer daily, preferably with a meal. For children 2 - 4 years of age, chew one-half (1/2) wafer daily.

Other Ingredients: Sucrose, Hydrogenated Cottonseed Oil, Vegetable Cellulose. Contains <2% of: Natural Orange Flavor, Silica, Vegetable Magnesium Stearate.

WARNING: If you are pregnant, nursing, taking any medications, planning any medical or surgical procedure or have any medical condition, consult your doctor before use. Discontinue use and consult your doctor if any adverse reactions occur. This product requires adult supervision and is not to be dispensed by children. Store at room temperature. Do not use if seal under cap is broken or missing.

KEEP OUT OF REACH OF CHILDREN
No Artificial Color or Flavor, No Milk, No Lactose, No Gluten, No Wheat, No Yeast, No Fish, Sodium Free.

100 Chewable $27.95

Order from: VitaGuardKeto.com

Vita-Guard Acidophilus

As a supplement, acidophilus is available as capsules, tablets, wafers, powders and a vaginal suppository. In addition to use as a supplement, acidophilus is found in some dairy products, such as yogurt, and is commercially added to many foods.

People commonly take acidophilus to treat a type of vaginal inflammation (bacterial vaginosis) and digestive disorders, as well as to promote the growth of good bacteria.

Acidophilus supports a favorable environment for the absorption of nutrients, encourages intestinal microflora balance, and maintains the healthy functioning of the intestinal system.** Intestinal microflora imbalance may lead to inefficient digestion.** Each strawberry flavored, milk-free chewable wafer contains one billion microorganisms at the time of manufacture.

Supplement Facts

Serving Size 1 Wafer

Amount Per Serving% Daily Value

Total Carbohydrate 1 g <1%**Sugars 1 g ***

Lactobacillus Blend 5 mg *** (which contains 1 billion active Lactobacillus Acidophilus Bifidobacterium Lactis at the time of manufacture)**Percent Daily Values are based on a 2,000 calorie diet.***Daily Value not established

.**Directions:** For adults, chew one (1) wafer three times daily, with or without meals.

Other Ingredients: Sucrose, Fructose, Vegetable Cellulose, Vegetable Stearic Acid. Contains <2% of: Citric Acid, Natural Flavors, Silica, Vegetable Magnesium Stearate. Providing one billion microorganisms per wafer at time of manufacture.

WARNING: If you are pregnant, nursing, taking any medications or have any medical condition, consult your doctor before use. Discontinue use and consult your doctor if any adverse reactions occur. Keep out of reach of children. Store unopened container at room temperature. Refrigerate after opening. Do not use if seal under cap is broken or missing. Suitable for Vegetarians.

100 Chewable $21.95

Order from: VitaGuardKeto.com

Moringa Oleifera Super Food

Moringa oleifera Is Very Nutritious

Protein: 2 grams

Vitamin B6: 19% of the RDA

Vitamin C: 12% of the RDA

Iron: 11% of the RDA

Riboflavin (B2): 11% of the RDA

Vitamin A (from beta-carotene): 9% of the RDA

Magnesium: 8% of the RDA

Rich in Antioxidants

May Lower Blood Sugar Levels

May Reduce Inflammation

Can Lower Cholesterol

May Protect Against Arsenic Toxicity

Moringa has many important vitamins and minerals. The leaves have 7 times more vitamin C than oranges and 15 times more potassium than bananas. It also has calcium, protein, iron, and amino acids, which help your body heal and build muscle.

It is packed with antioxidants, substances that can protect cells from damage and may boost your immune system. There's some evidence that some of these antioxidants can also lower blood pressure and reduce fat in the blood and body.

120 Caplets $33.95

Order from: VitaGuardKeto.com

Ginkgo Biloba

Ginkgo helps to maintain peripheral circulation to the extremities.** In addition, Ginkgo helps support memory, especially occasional mild memory problems associated with aging.** Our Ginkgo Biloba consists of high-quality herbs standardized to contain 24% Ginkgo Flavone Glycosides.

Gingko Biloba is an herbal plant extract that is commonly used in Chinese medicine to fight a variety of illnesses and diseases. It's best known for improving brain health and is often taken by people who are hoping to improve their mental and cognitive health. Many people aren't away of the other physical benefits of this herb. It can help treat pain, blood disorders, mood disorders and more. Improves Cognitive Health, Improved Dementia Symptoms, Fights Anxiety, Fights PMS Symptoms, Improves Libido, Treats Migraines, Improves Sleep, Fights Fibromyalgia.

Supplement Facts: Serving Size 1 Softgel, % Daily Value , Ginkgo Biloba Extract 60 mg ** . (standardized to contain 24% . Ginkgo Flavone Glycosides, 14.4 mg) . **Daily Value not established.

Directions: For adults, take one (1) softgel twice daily, preferably with meals. No Artificial Flavor or Sweetener, No Preservatives, No Sugar, No Starch, No Milk, No Lactose,

No Gluten, No Wheat, No Yeast, No Fish, Sodium Free.

100 Capsules $27.95

Order from: VitaGuardKeto.com

Conclusion

Find a Vita-Guard Keto Class You Can Join

The number of Vita-Guard Keto classes are growing across the nation. These classes will help you with your Keto journey. You may request a location by sending an email to: vitaguardketo1912@gmail.com.

A Final Word About the Keto Foods

Don't try to switch from your regular diet to the Keto diet too fast. Try new dishes each week and acquire the taste.

Take Your Vita-Guard Keto Regularly

Remember to take one in the morning and one in the

evening.

Drink plenty of fluids

You may need to drink a sports drink, Gatorade or Pedia-lyte to replace electrolytes caused from weight loss.

Should you have questions about Vita-Guard Keto or about your weight loss program, we are your personal coach. Contact us at email: vitaguard1912@gmail.com. Or, go to the website www.vitaguardketo.com.

www.ingramcontent.com/pod-product-compliance
Lightning Source LLC
Chambersburg PA
CBHW061819250726
48657CB00001B/503